SOMATIC YOGA

FOR NERVOUS SYSTEM REGULATION

41 Guided Techniques To Overcome Chronic
Stress & Strengthen Your Mind-Body Connection
In Just 10 Minutes A Day

689 Burke Rd
Camberwell Victoria 3124
Australia

www.LearnWellBooks.com

We're led by God. Our business is also committed to supporting kids' charities. At the time of printing, we have donated well over $100,000 to enable mentoring services for underprivileged children. By choosing our books, you are helping children who desperately need it. Thank you.

This Is Really Important.
It's a Sincere Thank You.

My name is Wayne, the founder of LearnWell.

My Dad put a book in my hands when I was 13. It was written by Zig Ziglar and it changed the course of my life. Since then, it's been books that have helped me get over breakups, learn how to be a good friend, study the lives of good people and books have been the source of my persistence through some pretty challenging times.

My purpose is now to return the favor. To create books that might be the turning point in the lives of people around the world, just like they've been for me. It's enough to almost bring me to tears to think of you holding this book, seeking information and wisdom from something that I've helped to create. I'm moved in a way that I can't fully explain.

We're a small and 'beyond-enthusiastic' team here at LearnWell. We're writers, editors, researchers, designers, formatters (oh ... and a bookkeeper!) who take your decision to learn with us incredibly seriously. We consider it a privilege to be part of your learning journey. Thank you for allowing us to join you.

If there's anything we did really well, anything we messed up, or anything AT ALL that we could do better, would you please write to us and tell us (like, right now!) We would love to hear from you!

readers@learnwellbooks.com

We're sending you our thanks, our love and our very best wishes.

Wayne

and the team at LearnWell Books.

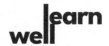

LearnWell Books

At LearnWell, we think learning is the most important thing a person can do. Learners grow, lead, and solve important problems. We consider it a privilege that you've chosen one of our books to learn from.

In return, we have invested significant effort in creating what we believe are the best books in the world, on the topics we choose to write about.

WORKBOOK

Accompanying this book is a comprehensive Workbook that will enhance your learning and increase your knowledge retention.

Before reading, please get your copy of the Workbook here:

www.learnwellbooks.com/breathe

It contains exercises that match the content of each chapter. It's interactive, user-friendly and proven to be the best way to absorb the valuable information in this book.

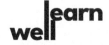

For You

I want you to feel at home in
your body, safe in your own mind,
and free in the world.

CONTENTS

WORKBOOK

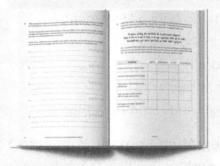

The average reader remembers just 14% of what they read. To dramatically enhance the amount of knowledge you absorb on this important topic, we have produced a user-friendly Workbook that follows the content of this book, chapter by chapter. Before beginning this book, make sure you receive a copy of your Workbook. Follow the link below:

Get Access To Your Free Workbook Here:

www.learnwellbooks.com/breathe

INTRODUCTION

The grip of chronic stress can suffocate the joy out of life. It can leave your nervous system running in overdrive until, eventually, it's in shambles. Feeling calm and at ease can become a distant memory you might fear will never be a reality again. After all, life doesn't slow down for anyone, so how can you possibly stay afloat?

Your nervous system is delicate, but it is also very receptive. It's always desperately searching for signs that you are safe enough to rest. You can offer it those signs.

Somatic yoga is a harmonious practice that is all about sending the right signals. It's a communication tool that teaches you how to speak your body's language. When you can speak that language, your nervous system can finally receive the message that's been lost in translation—you are safe enough to heal.

I used to carry burdens that were so heavy my nervous system began to buckle. I was plagued with panic attacks that would send me running to the ER, anxiety that followed me like a cloud, and heaps of unresolved trauma. As a trained yoga teacher, I couldn't understand why I couldn't shake these problems. I didn't carry the calm you would expect from someone who practiced yoga and meditated every day.

But there was one crucial mistake that was keeping my nervous system dysregulated. It allowed my stress to outweigh my efforts until I wasn't just anxious, I was sick. Along my recovery path,

I started a somatic practice that pulled everything together. It revealed the flaws in the way I was practicing yoga. And it's why I'm here sharing somatic yoga with you.

Whether you're trying yoga for the first time or you're an experienced practitioner wanting to deepen your practice, this book is for you. Let me save your nervous system the effort, and let's get straight to the point. Your mind and body are more connected than you will ever know. Somatic yoga is an all-encompassing, embodied practice that can treat chronic stress from the body to the mind. It leaves no stone unturned.

Learning the movements of this powerful practice is only a fraction of somatic yoga. The movements are what you see from the outside. But inside, the practice is expansive and deeply healing. It is nourishing for the entire nervous system: mind, body, and spirit.

To start you off with the understanding you need for a successful somatic practice, in the first four chapters, I'm going to offer you some valuable information about yoga, somatic practice, and how to get started. These will include:

 Chapter 1: A breakdown of why and how somatic yoga can regulate the nervous system.

 Chapter 2: All about the nervous system, including how it works and how it runs your life.

 Chapter 3: How to set up a nervous system nurturing practice space for your routine.

Chapter 4: The science behind how somatic yoga can fast-track your healing and bring you a lasting sense of calm.

Once you're confident and ready to jump into the exercises, you will find 41 effective somatic yoga exercises split across the next 5 chapters. They will include:

 Chapter 5: Exercises and poses for stress reduction and relaxation.

 Chapter 6: Practices to enhance your body awareness with mindfulness.

 Chapter 7: Bends, twists, and turns for flexibility and mobility.

 Chapter 8: Challenging poses for balance and coordination.

 Chapter 9: Poses to find strength and stability within your body.

 Chapter 10: Techniques to integrate the mind and body.

Then, to finish this book on the best note and start your somatic practice, Chapter 11 will guide you through the process of creating your own 10-minute somatic yoga routine. Ten minutes a day is enough to build a foundation of calm within your nervous system.

So, if you're tired of being stressed, fatigued, and highly strung, join me as we remember to breathe, move, and heal. I'm honored to guide you through this learning process, and I can't wait to see you come out the other side refreshed to your deepest inner self.

Love, Rose

1

BREATHE
MOVE
HEAL

Why Somatic Yoga Is The Answer
To Nervous System Dysregulation

*"The rhythm of the body, the melody of the mind
and the harmony of the soul create the symphony
of life."*

– B.K.S. Iyengar

The smell of coffee pierced the air as I stood in line at my local grocer's in-store cafe. It was a smell I normally enjoyed. However, the strength of it, coupled with my other overexcited senses, made my heart start to pound. Shopping trolleys rattled along the floor, there was a toddler throwing a tantrum in aisle 6 and suddenly, I could hear the air vents roaring. Being sucked into the present moment had never felt so jarring.

I tried to breathe as the barista placed my coffee on the counter. Forcing a smile, I tapped my card against the machine, dropped a coin into the tip jar, and made for the door. From the outside, I must have seemed in a rush to be somewhere, but nobody would have guessed that it was the closest bathroom stall. I stood in the cubicle behind a closed door, gasping while I clutched my beating chest. Anxiety had me gripped between its cold, bony fingers.

Not one thing in particular had happened to trigger this episode. It had been a good day. I'd just been to the gym, eaten a solid meal, and done my shopping for the week. One minute, I'm looking forward to a grande cappuccino, next minute, I've got enough adrenaline to tackle a bear.

Sure, the lights were bright, the noise was a lot, and mild anxiety was sort of my default at the time. But these episodes would happen too often, out of the blue, and without any sort of pattern between them. They slowly developed into an anxiety disorder, and I felt powerless.

When the words "disorder" or "chronic" pop up, we generally assume it means life-long. We assume that once a condition has progressed to a certain level, there's little turning back. We may do all the things we know to help and still feel stuck. And when that happens, these words can become a crutch to explain why our healing can't go any further.

Whether that's a chronic psychiatric disorder like anxiety or depression or something physical like sciatica or fatigue, the principle is the same. These are things we are often prepared by the medical system to live with rather than live through. If this sounds anything like you, you've come to the right place.

While I didn't understand what was causing my anxiety disorder at the time, now, years later, I do. The chronic stress of the life I was living, constantly working hard, thinking my way through problems, and pushing onward through heaps of unresolved trauma, kept my body in fight-or-flight mode.

My nervous system was brittle.

Rather than a tight set of nylon strings, able to bounce off any stress, my nervous system was a stick of dry spaghetti. One wrong move and snap! Everything I thought was helping me cope, like extensive talk therapy and cardio, was actually adding pressure to my nervous system. But the nervous system doesn't get stronger with more pressure. It becomes overloaded until it breaks down.

The key to strengthening the nervous system lies in gentle re-engagement following stress. It takes time and slowness, and it requires an improved mind-body connection. This is where somatic yoga can be a pivotal addition to your life.

I'd already practiced yoga regularly up until this story, which formed part of my coping strategy at the time. However, I didn't see it as a deeply healing modality for the nervous system but rather as another way to release energy and stay healthy. That was until I discovered somatic experiencing after a traumatic life event, and everything came together.

Somatic experiencing focuses on gentle movements with the sole intention of nervous system regulation and trauma release. It taps into our body's natural regulating mechanisms, improving wellness for both body and mind simultaneously. It's often referred to as a body-up approach.

I continued to practice somatic exercises daily as a compliment to the training I was doing to become a yoga teacher. Without a conscious effort, the practices began to merge. My yoga practice deepened in such a profound way that it was as if I experienced the true power of yoga for the first time. It wasn't long before those almost daily anxiety attacks became weekly, monthly, and then few and far between. The word "disorder" faded from my vocabulary.

What was once a matter of flexibility of the body became flexibility of the mind as well. Rather than anxiously completing my daily yoga set, desperate to see improvements in my health, I was able to let go. I surrendered to the process and began to truly *feel* my way through healing.

This process caught me by surprise as I started being able to sit in stillness for the first time ever without my mind racing. No background TV shows, radio, or someone to talk to. I could simply be present without the constant need to be somewhere, do something, or distract myself from the inner turmoil that used to be normal for me.

Somatic yoga is the marriage of two unbelievably powerful movement-based healing modalities. They fit so well together because they've already been merged in many ways for thousands of years. While somatic practice is a relatively new modality, it's something that has informally been a part of many ancient healing modalities – now we simply have a word for it.

In this chapter, I'll explain everything you need to know to understand somatic yoga, where it comes from, and how it works. I'll also answer the questions, "Well, what's the difference between normal yoga and somatic yoga?" and "Isn't yoga somatic anyway?" I'm so excited to share this practice with you and guide your transformation with the help of this book.

 If you feel it necessary to get started with the exercises right away, you will find the first set of somatic yoga exercises in Chapter 5. However, I will encourage you to invest some energy in reading the theory section of this book to ensure that your knowledge base supports a successful practice. Without an understanding of why you're doing certain movements, you might not lean into them in the way your nervous system truly needs.

This isn't a "works for some but not for others" approach. Somatic yoga works because it nourishes the nervous system. No matter who you are, where you're from, or how many years you've been on this earth, our nervous systems all have the same wiring. We all have a beautiful brain and a body that can feel. That's all you need to see tremendous progress in your healing and wellness journey. So, if you're ready, come along with me, and let's get started.

THE ORIGINS OF SOMATIC YOGA

Yoga is the science and art of healthy living. It is more than a simple physical practice; it is the pursuit of harmony between mind and body dating back to 2700 BC.[1] Its positions, poses, and stretches are only a gateway to higher states of health, living, and consciousness. This is because they activate the nervous system in ways that promote well-being.

The practice has always had deep roots in mindfulness and body awareness, with Western society shifting the focus predominantly onto physical health. Think hot yoga, power yoga, and stretching for flexibility purposes. However, with the prevalence of chronic stress in our modern world and all the related symptoms and disease, it's time to shift the focus back to a more inward-focused yoga practice.

Somatic yoga is the embodiment of mind-body harmony. It is the reemergence of yoga's mindful roots along with the modern understanding of the somatic experience we have cultivated in recent years. It enhances the health of both mind and body simultaneously.

Philosopher Thomas Hanna was the neurology researcher who pioneered the term "somatic" in the late 1960s. Upon coming to understand that every psychological process occurs alongside changes in the body's systems, he realized that problems within the psyche must be addressed with the help of the body – through the mind-body connection. He referred to this interconnected system as a "soma." In Greek, the word soma means "the living body in its wholeness."[2]

Soon, as somatic practice became increasingly popular for its positive impact on nervous system health, many yoga practitioners realized its connection to yoga philosophy. The two modalities met to become a new and increasingly effective healing modality: somatic yoga.

PRINCIPLES OF SOMATIC YOGA

When the mind experiences stress, the body responds by activating the fight-flight-or-freeze nervous system state. With the best intentions, the body tries to protect us from stress by bracing us for it. We will discuss the nervous system in more depth in Chapter 2, but for now, all you need to understand is that experiencing this response creates distance between the mind and body.

The stress response is an uncomfortable experience of increased tension. This tension can manifest in various ways depending on your nervous system. In the long term, it leads to posture, balance, and strength disequilibrium. This often creates or contributes to chronic pain and anxiety. Your nervous system becomes chronically dysregulated as the tension is left unresolved and builds into dis-ease and discomfort.

When the body is uncomfortable, the mind can't feel safe and will withdraw or react in a way that further perpetuates this nervous system response. The cycle continues until you actively break it. However, once the tension has manifested in the body from anxiety, trauma, degradation, or injury, it's not something the mind can solve—at least not on its own.

The mind and body must solve problems within their combined system in unison.

Somatic yoga works with a set of principles that combine into an embodiment practice that will empower you to heal bidirectionally. That means you will heal the mind using the body and the body with the mind simultaneously. These principles come together to nourish the nervous system in a balanced and sustainable way. They include:

Mindfulness

During a somatic yoga practice, you will engage and center your mind through deep and rhythmic breathing. You will be encouraged to bring your awareness into the present moment inside your body, become aware of all its sensations, and mindfully move to meet your body's needs.

Body Awareness

Somatic yoga includes some of the fundamental somatic exercises combined with yoga positions. One of the most important somatic practices is the body scan, which encourages improved body awareness. This practice focuses on the sensory experience of your body and its movements. Improved body awareness will help you pinpoint problem areas and patterns to release more effectively and find relief.

Intention

As you move, stretch, and hold your body in new ways, you will be encouraged to set intentions for your movements. Your intentions will align with your desired outcome and unique problem areas. For example:

- You might choose to move with the intention of releasing stored trauma, allowing your body to repeat movements more rigorously, shake, or move as needed to let go.

- You might choose to focus on relaxation, allowing your movements to slow and soften in a way that is soothing for both body and mind.

- You might set the intention to enliven more energy within your system, moving and stretching in ways that get your blood flowing and bring you joy.

There are endless possibilities for what you can achieve with somatic yoga through intention. Your intention will govern how you approach exercises and will ensure your mind remains an active guide in the process.

Empowerment

As you experience somatic yoga and become familiar with the first three principles, you will come to feel a life-changing sense of empowerment. This practice is all about learning to listen to the body's language – feeling.

With an increased mind-body awareness, you will come to understand what your body has been trying to tell you through the pain, stiffness, and tension. Once you can hear it, somatic yoga will help you trust it so that you can feel empowered to nurture your own healing.

SOMATIC YOGA VS. TRADITIONAL YOGA

Before we move on, I'd like to make a clear distinction between somatic yoga and traditional yoga. While true traditional yoga does include many of the aspects of somatic yoga, it is generally more focused on postures, alignment, balance, and all the physical aspects involved. The sense of relaxation and centeredness you might experience is more of a secondary benefit, particularly in the Western practice of traditional yoga.

Somatic yoga takes the stress-relieving benefits of yoga to a new level by focusing on its introspective aspects. It's less about moving your body to fit the postures and more about adjusting postures to fit your body's needs. It's still important to keep good posture and re-educate your body into more beneficial movement patterns, but somatic yoga does so in a way that is nurturing, releasing, and more embodied.

Where you might hold a rigid pose in traditional yoga for a count of 3 breaths, the same pose in somatic yoga might include gentle swaying, rocking, and deeper, more intentional breathing. Your intuition is encouraged to help move your body within the postures and stretches in ways that feel good to you. This freedom is what allows your nervous system to fully regulate itself, calming the mind and making your body a safer place to be.

The nervous system is a complex system that spans your entire body and includes the brain.[3] It impacts both your mental and physical states at any given time. Understanding how it works and why somatic yoga can influence it in such positive and lasting ways will make this practice so much more effective for your healing.

this is very helpful

When you're ready, turn the page to Chapter 2, and let's explore how the nervous system works, why it's related to stress and relaxation, and how somatic yoga can effectively regulate it. You don't need to wait months to find relief. Practicing somatic yoga with the proper understanding will help you tap into your body's natural regulating mechanisms for an often instant sense of relief.

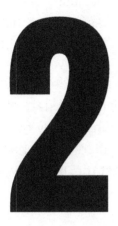

HOW YOUR
NERVOUS SYSTEM
RUNS YOUR LIFE

And How To Regain Control Of Both

"The nervous system controls and regulates every function of the body, and yoga is a powerful tool to keep it in balance."

– Elena Brower

The curtains swayed in the midnight breeze as my peripherals caught every movement. Thoughts of the day ahead spiraled around as I tried to catch the moments of peace in between. Nothing major was happening in the morning, just work. But my body responded to the day ahead as if it was a milestone I was underprepared for.

In this moment, desperate to sleep, I felt a prisoner in my body. There was no sense of control over my heightened state of mind, and it seemed my body did not care for what I truly needed. If you've ever had sleepless nights, you'll understand when I say that it felt like my body was working against me. In reality, it was me who wasn't working with my body.

Regaining control of your life starts with learning to understand the body's language. The body speaks in sensations, tension, emotions, and movements. It doesn't respond to thoughts; it responds to the embodiment of those thoughts.

When I was wishing my body into a restful state every night, I wasn't embodying rest and relaxation. And even when I was trying to, by the time my body decided that work the next day was too much of a threat to get sleep, the game was already over. It had already given me ample warnings and requests and now it couldn't trust me. Looking back, I can recognize the attempts my body made to communicate stress throughout the day. I just wasn't listening.

Only once I started forming a better relationship with my body did I start to hear its whispers. I could feel my shoulders tighten before a meeting. I could sense the shift in my emotions as I sat waiting in the morning traffic. The subtle communications

The body speaks in sensations, tension, emotions, and movements. It doesn't respond to thoughts; it responds to the embodiment of those thoughts.

of soreness, stiffness, and frustration were all there. Ignoring my needs in those moments led me to the point of no return, staring at the ceiling until 3 am almost every night.

As you learn to tune into your body throughout this book, you will realize that by the time your body is taking you prisoner, there has already been an entire missed conversation within your nervous system. Somatic yoga is a practice that will allow you to translate what's being said and meet your body's needs for a more regulated nervous system and a more regulated life.

Instead of feeling trapped in your body, you will learn to make friends with it. Understanding the nervous system and how it impacts your daily life will give you the insight you need to start feeling your way into better states of being rather than wishing them in. Join me now as we uncover how the nervous system functions, why it's the reason your body is stuck in a state of chronic stress, and how somatic yoga can soothe it into lasting regulation.

OVERVIEW OF THE NERVOUS SYSTEM

The nervous system is like a circuit board with many switches. Made up of a complex network of nerves, the spinal cord, and the brain, it expands across the entire body, waiting for signals to be switched on and off to keep the body in balance. It's a delicate system that relies on the appropriate movement of energy to stay functioning as it should.

Some of the switches that can signal changes in your nervous system include your breath, movement, emotions, and environment. These can trigger vital changes required for health and well-being.

As soon as your nervous system registers a signal, such as a change in breath, a strong emotion, or an external threat, it can flip from one state to another in response. For example, if you've ever taken a couple of deep breaths to calm yourself down after a stressful event, you used your breath to change the state of your nervous system.

There are three elementary nervous system states, known as rest-and-digest, fight-or-flight, and freeze. Fight, flight, and freeze are all sympathetic nervous system responses, and rest-and-digest is a parasympathetic nervous system response.[4]

The sympathetic nervous system is like a circuit breaker, protecting the body from overload. It activates as a threat response in an attempt to protect you from perceived danger. When it activates, your breathing may quicken, your heart rate may rise, and you may experience the anxiety needed to escape, fight, or fawn from the threat.

However, chronic stress can cause constant perceived danger, which creates a dysregulated sympathetic nervous system response. This is when the fight-flight-or-freeze response becomes the default, and the body becomes stuck in survival mode.

THE CONNECTION BETWEEN STRESS, RELAXATION, AND YOUR BODY

The body's natural state of homeostasis is the parasympathetic rest-and-digest state.[5] This is when your muscles can ease up, your stomach can unknot, and your mind feels calm. It relies on a sense of safety within yourself and your environment to become active.

A regulated nervous system doesn't mean that your body never experiences its sympathetic response. Regulation in the nervous system means that it can easily flip between states when necessary without becoming stuck for too long in one or the other. It functions as intended and can maintain its calm parasympathetic state as long as there is no real threat.

For example, when a stressor occurs, like someone swerving toward your car while driving, your heart rate might elevate, your body might sweat, and your thoughts might race. But as soon as the threat has passed and you get a moment to breathe, your nervous system should bounce back to a more relaxed state quickly and fully.

The trouble is when your nervous system is chronically dysregulated, it can become difficult to flip the switch into rest-and-digest after a threat has occurred. You might also notice your nervous system perceiving more situations and events as threats, even when they're not.

Just like my anxiety disorder and insomnia, my nervous system had become so dysregulated from chronic stress that its sympathetic response would activate when I least expected it to. It would respond in a big way to small stressors, and I would struggle to get myself back to rest-and-digest.

When your nervous system is dysregulated, your sympathetic response is either overactive or underactive. An overactive sympathetic nervous system response is responsible for anxiety, panic, and an urgency to either escape the situation or stay and fight. An underactive sympathetic response can cause you to freeze into a state of shutdown, where your emotions become numb, your body slows down, and your mind becomes blank.

Being in these states for too long and too often can cause all sorts of problems as your body prioritizes energy for immediate survival. That's why common problems associated with chronic stress include:

- Digestive issues
- Weakened immune function
- Muscle tension
- Chronic pain
- Anxiety
- Panic attacks

- Inflammation
- Fatigue
- Headaches
- Sleep disturbances
- Lack of concentration
- Memory problems
- Depression

These are all serious symptoms that, if ignored, can lead to long-term illness and disease.[6] The good news is that as quickly as your nervous system can become dysregulated, somatic yoga can restore balance.

A dysregulated nervous system needs to be re-educated into regulation. This takes a consistent relaxation practice to remind your nervous system what safety feels like. Just as chronic stress slowly causes the fight-flight-or-freeze response to become default, a practice like somatic yoga can encourage the nervous system to choose rest-and-digest instead.

HOW SOMATIC YOGA BENEFITS NERVOUS SYSTEM REGULATION

Somatic yoga is an impactful practice that can heal nervous system dysregulation because it works to reinforce the switches that signal safety in the body. It allows you to take control of the things you can to influence your default nervous system state. Some of the practices that form part of somatic yoga, which stimulate the rest-and-digest response and regulate the nervous system, include:

Breathwork

Breathwork encompasses much more than just deep breathing. There are specific controlled breathing patterns and methods that you will learn in this book, which have been proven to balance the nervous system in minutes. Controlled breathing can slow the heart rate, focus the mind, and reestablish normal oxygen levels in the thinking part of the brain rather than the brain's fear-centers.[7]

Mindful Movement

Mindful movement is a way for us to release energy and nourish the body through movement while practicing mindfulness. It enhances our mind-body awareness so that we can better feel and identify the signals our body sends. The better we can recognize the signals that trigger both relaxation and fight-flight-or-freeze, the better we can intercept a sympathetic nervous system response and strengthen the parasympathetic response for a regulated nervous system.[8]

Humming And Vocalisation

An important set of nerves that run through the body is known collectively as the vagus nerve. This nerve system is responsible for the parasympathetic response. The stronger it is, the more safe, calm, and clear you can feel.

Activating the vagus nerve is one of the most effective and almost instant ways to regulate the nervous system. And because it runs down the neck alongside the vocal cords, their vibrations can stimulate it for a quick parasympathetic response.[9]

Somatic yoga will include exercises that use humming or sound vibrations to help stimulate the vagus nerve and contribute to its health.

Body Scanning

While many of the practices, such as breathwork and humming, can offer quick relief from stressful states of mind and body, it's important to build a healthier relationship with your body for the long term. Body scanning is a technique that is fundamental to somatic yoga and is something that sets it apart from traditional yoga. This is because it is a practice that asks you to tune into your body, identify areas of tension, stiffness, or anxiety, and sit with them.

Body scanning is not about trying to escape discomfort. It trains your mind to identify discomfort without judgment so that you can meet the needs causing the discomfort rather than shrug it off. Learning to sit with your body through discomfort builds resilience to stress.

However, this practice also asks you to identify areas of softness, relaxation, and joy to better identify and recall these ideal states. Body scanning builds a stronger picture of what relaxation feels like so that safety becomes more accessible.[10] You will have the opportunity to learn how to complete a full body scan in Chapter 6.

The state of your nervous system will determine how you show up in the world. It will impact how much you sleep, socialize, eat, and think. It will also determine how you feel about yourself and how comfortable your body is. A nervous system with poor vagal tone can leave you on edge, unhappy, and hopeless. But you can control the switches that decide which nervous system state is your default.

If your lifestyle is chaotic, you've experienced trauma, or you're not sure why you're anxious all the time, your nervous system is likely in need of a tune-up. Like a guitar, the nylon strings of your nervous system become weak and toneless, and they're not going to tune themselves.

To take control of your life and feel a sense of internal safety, you need to actively practice techniques that will get your strings strumming harmonious melodies again. If you're ready to start tuning into your body and find the relief you're looking for, turn the page to Chapter 3, where we will discuss the essentials of starting a somatic practice.

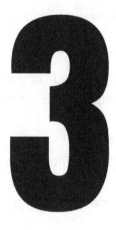

BEGIN WITH
SPACE AND MIND

**Your Best Set-Up
For Somatic Success**

*"We should all find a quiet place, a peaceful space,
to bury the chaos and rest for a while."*

– Christy Ann Martine

If you've ever had someone give you a gift out of spite or force, you will understand how the intention behind an action determines its impact. This same concept can apply to everything you do. For example, moving with urgency looks and feels very different than moving with grace and softness, and it will impact your nervous system state.

In yoga, it's believed that everything is a part of the practice. How you carry yourself in every moment of your life is yoga. That's why it's seen as an embodiment practice.

This boils down to one key rule for a stress-free life:

 The way you do things matters.

For your somatic yoga practice to be effective, it's important that you take time to integrate it into your life in a full and embodied way. Imagine trying to reach a state of relaxation in the midst of rush hour traffic or sitting down and quieting your mind with a TV blaring in the background. Your environment is a vital element to a successful somatic yoga practice.

However, your environment is not limited to your external space. It includes your internal thoughts, beliefs, and emotions. Just like receiving a gift charged with resentment, your mindset about somatic yoga will permeate its effectiveness. This chapter will help ensure that your mindset is charged with intentions that will guarantee a great somatic yoga experience.

Before moving on to the exercises, take this opportunity to learn how to better integrate somatic yoga into your life and heart so that you can get the most out of it. In this chapter, we will explore all the ways you can create a safe space for your body and mind to immerse yourself in the joy and peace that comes with a successful somatic yoga session.

SETTING INTENTIONS AND CREATING A SAFE SPACE

Our minds are constantly being shaped by the world around us, our experiences, and our behavior patterns. Left to its own devices, the mind can run with thoughts that don't serve us, trigger negative emotions and behaviors based on past events, and subsequently create the reality we see.

Without a clear direction, it's difficult for the mind to remember what we have set out to achieve. That's where setting intentions is a vital practice needed for success in any area of your life. What you set out to do is the start of getting things done. With conscious effort and control over our intentions, they can push the limits of our lives and make room for bigger and better experiences.

Intentions stretch our beliefs of what's possible. And when the mind believes something is possible, it's two steps closer to experiencing it.[11]

Your Internal Environment

Sometimes, a simple intention is so powerful that it alone can attract the experience, even without much further action. For example, one of my favorite intentions to repeat every morning before I start my daily somatic yoga session is

 I embody joy.

Sometimes, just saying this intention out loud warms my heart and puts a smile on my face. It's that powerful.

Intentions don't have to be paragraphs of things we want to achieve. They can be simple, powerful, and easy. Whatever you want to call into your reality during your somatic yoga session can become the intention you set. Some examples of intentions that work well with somatic yoga include:

- I feel safe within my body.

- My body is a temple. Every cell in it is alive and healthy.

- Peace comes naturally to me.

- I release any tension within my body.

- Today I choose love over fear.

- My joints move freely and without pain.

- All emotions are welcome today. I honor how I feel.

- I move with softness.

- Life is abundant and I'm tapped into it..

- I embody joy.

- My nervous system knows peace.

 The easiest way to come up with an intention is to think about what state of being you'd like to achieve with your practice. This could be an emotion, a mindset, or a level of comfort. Find the word, then add "I embody X" or "Today X comes easily to me." You'll know when you've found an intention that works when saying it creates an emotional shift in you. A good intention directly impacts the success and enjoyment of your practice. Take some time to answer the questions in your Workbook to make finding an intention easier.

You can choose a new intention for each somatic yoga session, or you can work with the same one for some time to really reinforce it. Once you've chosen your intention, try to embody it. Imagine what it would be like to experience what you're hoping for. How would your body feel? What expression would be on your face? Which emotions would present themselves? Allow these experiences to grow as you allow them in.

Your External Environment

Now that you've practiced setting up your internal environment let's discuss ways you can bring yoga into your external environment. Your external environment will include where you choose to practice somatic yoga. Of course, you can certainly use these practices at any time in any space when needed, but it helps to have a dedicated place where you actively practice somatic yoga to give your nervous system a sense of safety and sameness.

To create a dedicated yoga space, you can:

- Pick somewhere you love in your home or even in nature.

- Set out a yoga mat or another surface with a steady grip.

- Add mood lighting to the area, like dimmable lights, salt lamps, or candles.

- Play relaxing music like meditative flute music or nature sounds.

- Add other sensory elements like a soft blanket, essential oils, or artwork you love.

- Eliminate distractions in this area. For example, make the space a "no phone zone."

Your practice environment should feel soothing to your nervous system. Each of these elements can help to bring down the stress response and encourage regulation. Make use of your senses, keep it simple, and build a practice space that feels good to you.

Having a dedicated, safe space to practice yoga where you know you won't be disturbed and can fully let go will deepen your practice tremendously. It's also a great way to find safety in a world that can feel chaotic. When you practice somatic yoga in a dedicated space every day, that space becomes sacred and can offer you comfort in times of stress. Even if you're not in the mood to practice, you can enter your space and address what's bothering you in a safe and effective way.

Safety is what the nervous system craves. Attaining it is its ultimate function. That's why doing things that help set you up for feelings of relaxation and joy works so well to reduce stress and regulate your nervous system. When your internal environment is aligned with a healthier objective, and you have a space where you know you can safely work towards that objective, your nervous system can relax.

PREPARING YOUR BODY AND MIND FOR SOMATIC YOGA

To get the most out of your somatic yoga practice, it helps to prepare your body and mind in various ways. Create a routine that you follow with each session to enhance your body's readiness for relaxation and stress relief. This will allow your nervous system to start receiving the signals for rest-and-digest before you've even started.

A great somatic yoga routine might look like:

1. Step 1: Getting into comfortable clothing and pouring a glass of water.

2. Step 2: Rolling out your yoga mat and setting the mood with scented candles and music.

3. Step 3: Sitting down on your mat and choosing an intention for the session.

4. Step 4: Checking in with yourself with 5 minutes of deep breathing and a body scan.

5. Step 5: Your choice of 3-5 somatic yoga poses and exercises.

6. Step 6: Remembering to repeat your intention throughout your practice.

7. Step 7: Checking back in with yourself for more breathing and meditation.

8. Step 8: Slowly closing the session by mindfully drinking some water, rolling up your mat, and blowing out the candles.

Remember, yoga is in the way you do everything. Letting it influence how you complete basic, everyday tasks will set you up for long-term nervous system regulation. Embody the softness and safety that you want to feel by moving more mindfully in everything you do. The benefits of somatic yoga don't start and end during a session; they carry over into your life and how you choose to live it.

As you practice, be sure to ground yourself into the present and create a nervous system-nourishing experience from the minute you roll out your mat. Somatic yoga is not about the movements themselves but rather their impact on your nervous system. There is an emphasis on the embodiment of peace, softness, and joy. But that comes easiest when you know how to tune in and listen to your body's needs in the moment.

If you're ready to maximize the calming effects of this practice instead of just going through the movements and wondering why they're not working, then come with me to the next chapter, where we will learn the essential building blocks of somatic yoga.

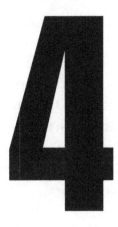

4

YOUR FASTEST PATH TO CALM

How To Maximize The Results
From Your Practice

*"The most important pieces of equipment you need
for doing yoga are your body and your mind."*

– Rodney Yee

Feeling my palms pressed firmly into the mat, I held my body in downward dog. Breathing deeply, I was going through the motions of my go-to daily yoga flow that had come together naturally after years of practicing. My mind was clear, my blood was flowing, and my form felt good. But I still went on to have a panic attack later that same day.

You see, something very important was missing from my practice. While I was practicing, I felt great, but the peace and stability yoga brought me ended when I rolled up my mat. I wasn't letting yoga spill over into the rest of my life the way an effective yoga practice should. The minute I was done, I'd reach for my phone to check my emails, and the stress would come rushing back.

That's where practicing somatic yoga changed everything.

Although my daily practice didn't look much different from the outside, I had opened up to new depths of regulation and joy. The somatic experience of yoga started to unfold emotional pain that was locked away in my body. It allowed the pent-up energy sitting in my muscles as chronic tension to shift and release.

But this didn't happen by continuing to go through the motions. I made a conscious effort to apply the principles of somatic yoga not only to my daily practice but also to my life. Because somatic yoga focuses on embodying the states of being you wish to achieve, those states start to become who you are. This is because they work to regulate your nervous system from the outside in – from the body up to the mind.

Using the movements and somatic strategies to deepen your mind-body awareness quickly tones your nervous system. A toned nervous system is a lasting state that will not undo easily, especially when you consistently reinforce its strength with daily somatic yoga. When done correctly, the movements and other elements come together to gently change the way you experience life. The benefits don't end when you roll up your mat. They stay with you, keeping your mind and body relaxed for hours.

As we discussed in Chapter 3, your nervous system reflects the states that it is most often in. When you are able to feel stable and relaxed for hours each day, your nervous system quickly becomes accustomed to safety and continues to operate from a state of regulation, even in the face of stress. Stress soon becomes a momentary experience, and calm becomes chronic.

To allow somatic yoga into your life as a part of who you are rather than what you do, let's go through the fastest path to calm and discuss all the ways that you can maximize your practice from the start. In this chapter, I'll be explaining the core somatic movements and how they work to enhance your overall nervous system state, why the way you breathe is essential, and how mindfulness ties everything together.

CORE SOMATIC MOVEMENTS AND THEIR PURPOSES

Traditional yoga will include many of the core somatic movements associated with somatic practice. However, as you practice somatic yoga, it will help to understand these key aspects to deepen your practice and increase awareness of their effectiveness. You might take more note of these experiences, purposefully lean into them, and witness the difference they make.

Dynamic Tension And Relaxation

Many of the somatic yoga movements work to release tension by making use of dynamic tension and relaxation. This is when the movements purposefully engage and tense a muscle and then shift into a release. The rhythmic contraction and relaxation cycle caused by dynamic tension and relaxation contributes to the release of chronic muscle tension and an improved stress response.

These basic repetitions demonstrate normal muscle function and regulate your nervous system by thoughtfully applying controlled stress to a muscle and offering relief. Eventually, the tension does not just release from muscle fatigue but from deep within the nervous system where it originates. This concept is also known as progressive muscle relaxation.[12] However, in somatic yoga, the practice is applied through movement.

Proprioceptive Neuromuscular Facilitation (PNF)

In somatic yoga, many of the stretches and positions work to engage the nervous system to reach and release tension that regular stretching won't achieve. One of the ways this is possible is with a technique called proprioceptive neuromuscular facilitation (PNF).

PNF works by engaging muscle groups in a complementary way to signal relaxation in the nervous system and release more tension. Many muscles work in pairs or groups to function. PNF leverages the relationships between muscles to deepen stretches quickly.[13]

For example, you are likely familiar with your 2 main upper arm muscles: the bicep and tricep. For the bicep to contract, the tricep must lengthen and relax, and vice versa. However, chronic tension can cause tight muscles that reduce mobility and inhibit proper muscle relaxation. PNF will include purposefully engaging and releasing the bicep muscle to deepen a tricep stretch. The bicep will release any pent-up tension that may be inhibiting the tricep stretch.

Stretching And Pandiculation

While somatic yoga does involve regular stretching as well as active stretching, where muscles are stretched into a position and deepened using the breath, it also includes pandiculation. Pandiculation is an active form of stretching that models nature's involuntary relaxation system.[14] Like a cat that stretches its body while yawning to prepare itself for being awake, we can access pandiculation on purpose to lengthen muscles without holding a passive stretching position.

I'll touch more on pandiculation in Chapter 6. But for now, all you need to know is that it is a powerful way to change the length and softness of muscles by retraining the nervous system. It is achieved by involving the brain in an active contraction of a muscle followed by a very slow melting release that leads to quick, easy, and long-lasting tension release.

Slow, Mindful, And Intuitive Movements

Unlike many other forms of yoga, which may involve breaking a sweat or holding difficult poses, somatic yoga is focused on your body and its needs. That's why movements are encouraged to be slow, soft, and mindful.

As we discussed in Chapter 2, moving mindfully means being aware of your body and moving in a focused and present way. This awareness improves your ability to recognize the signs of dysregulation and take steps to release tension and enter a more regulated state. Body scanning and other mindfulness practices are included in the mindfulness aspect of somatic yoga.

However, along with moving more mindfully, you may also incorporate some intuitive movements within the exercises. This means allowing your body to move and deepen into the positions and movements. For example, if swaying gently feels good in a forward bend, go with it! Or, if an exercise calls for 3 deep breaths, but you don't feel satisfied, keep breathing a little longer. The somatic part of somatic yoga means being in tune with your body and listening to what it needs.

Shaking And Neurogenic Tremors

An often misunderstood component of somatic practice is the involuntary muscle tremors that can occur. This is when the muscles start to shake or move without your control when holding the body in certain positions or angles. Although it might seem unusual or even a bit concerning, this mechanism is known as neurogenic tremors and is the body's natural way of releasing stress. A common example is when a prey animal escapes danger, it can almost always be seen quite literally shaking off the stress.[15]

Somatic yoga does not include the classic exercise that is designed to consciously induce this mechanism. However, because muscle fatigue is a big trigger for muscle tremors and shaking, you may experience a somatic release during your somatic yoga practice. Although you can easily stop muscle tremors by shifting out of a position, I will encourage you to ride them out for a moment. Doing so will allow your nervous system to get rid of excess stress and tension.

You might also feel intuitively drawn to shaking a body part during an exercise. For example, when completing somatic yoga leg lifts, you may try shaking out the leg after each round. This is just an additional somatic element you can add to your practice for further benefits.

The way you move and complete somatic yoga exercises is paramount to the effectiveness of your practice. The nervous system responds well to slow, intentional movements because the brain is a vital component of the nervous system. Involving it in a more mindful and conscious way will allow the movements to improve nervous system functioning.

Each of the exercises throughout the rest of this book has the potential to improve your proprioception and interoception, as they all work to build nervous system awareness and regulation.

Proprioception is your body's ability to understand where it is in space and how to move without your brain needing to think. For example, when you walk, your proprioception includes your balance, the consistent rhythm of your feet hitting the ground, and your arms swaying. It's what allows you to quickly duck when you walk under a branch or walk through a doorway without hitting the frame.

Interoception is the brain's ability to sense the internal state of your body and determine its needs. Every organ in your body has receptors that communicate sensations to your nervous system, which it can read and respond to. For example, without interoception, you wouldn't know when you needed the bathroom, when you were hungry, or when you were getting cold.

Somatic yoga improves all functions related to the nervous system by strengthening the mind-body connection and working to re-educate it into relaxation. But every exercise is tightly linked with another involuntary bodily function that you can learn to control for better nervous system tone – breathing.

INTEGRATING BREATH WITH MOVEMENT FOR ENHANCED AWARENESS

Integrating breath with movement means learning how to synchronize each inhale and exhale with various movements and intentions. The breath is a powerful tool in somatic yoga. Synchronizing breath with movement enhances the mind-body connection and makes you more receptive to your body's energy flow. Consciously controlling and focusing on the breath during movements quietens the mind for a much deeper sense of relaxation.

Somatic yoga encourages deep diaphragmatic breathing, which activates the parasympathetic nervous system. However, when combined with slow, intentional movements, the parasympathetic response is greatly reinforced. When the parasympathetic nervous system activates, heart rate slows, muscle tension releases, and blood pressure decreases.[16]

The breath also allows you to deepen stretches by triggering relaxation that reaches further into your muscles and joints for improved mobility, flexibility, and strength as it circulates oxygen around the body.

Integrating breath with movement is also known as building a breath-movement connection. A strong breath-movement connection builds resilience and improves trauma release as it offers another way for you to address and release painful emotions and memories.

There may be times during your somatic yoga practice when an uncomfortable emotion or memory surfaces. This is when you can use your breath-movement connection to acknowledge the experience gracefully, using the breath to explore it and let it go. With somatic yoga, you will learn how to pull your awareness deeper into thoughts, sensations, and tension as you inhale and how to release it on the exhale. This may come with time and practice, but another key element of somatic yoga will help bring it all together—mindfulness.

THE ROLE OF MINDFULNESS IN SOMATIC YOGA

My yoga practice was perfectly relaxing and enjoyable in the moment. I had learned about yoga's history and the many profound teachings that it encompasses, but I didn't allow its philosophy to unfold within me. I didn't embody yoga.

Embodiment of a somatic yoga practice requires you to look within and allow the shifts that present themselves to happen. Whether they carry discomfort, joy, or other symptoms of healing, they won't complete themselves without your acknowledgment and acceptance. You have to become an active participant in your healing, and that takes mindfulness.

Mindfulness and yoga should go together like a fish in water. However, many Western variations of yoga have lost the depth it is meant to possess. Somatic yoga is a way to reconnect the roots of yoga while simultaneously understanding the scientific significance of movements to our advantage. To integrate these two seemingly separate worlds, mindfulness must be at the foundation of your practice.

When you allow mindfulness to strengthen the significance of your daily somatic practice, deepen your relaxation response, and shift your nervous system state to chronic peace instead of stress, your entire life will reflect your practice. This is the essence of yoga.

So, as you continue on to the exercises that wait for you between chapters 5 and 9, let mindfulness always be step 1. A successful and fast path to calm requires your full commitment and attention. You need to be present with the exercises the minute your feet touch the mat. Then, when you roll it up at the end of your session, let your mind continue to explore peace in everything you do. Embody it, and you will become it.

When you're ready, there are 6 chapters filled with 41 essential somatic yoga exercises. Each chapter serves a specific purpose, allowing you to enjoy a single chapter as a full somatic yoga set. However, I invite you to take note of which exercises resonate with you the most so that they can form part of your personalized 10-minute somatic yoga practice that you will have the opportunity to create in Chapter 11.

5

STRESS REDUCTION
AND RELAXATION

"The paradox of relaxation is the renewal of the mind, rekindling of spirit, and revitalizing of strength."

– Lailah Gifty Akita

DIAPHRAGMATIC BREATHING

This exercise will accompany your somatic yoga practice. It is a powerful, nervous system-soothing practice on its own and a great relaxation tool for any occasion. Use this technique when asked to deepen your breath during an exercise.

We discussed the vagus nerve in Chapter 2 and how it runs alongside your vocal chords. However, it continues down to your diaphragm, below your lungs. Diaphragmatic breathing activates the parasympathetic nervous system response by expanding the lungs down into your diaphragm, which stimulates the vagus nerve. It is also known as deep belly breathing.

Instructions

To complete a round of diaphragmatic breathing, find a comfortable seated position with a good upright posture. If needed, you can also complete this exercise lying down on your back.

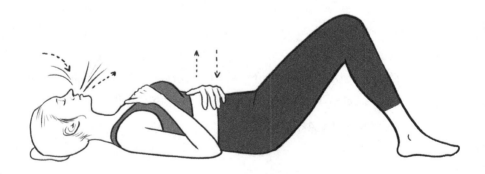

Step 1: Place your right hand on your chest and your left hand on your belly.

The hand positioning of this exercise helps build awareness of your breathing patterns. As you breathe, your right hand should stay still, and your left hand should gently rise as you fill your belly.

Step 2: Inhale Deeply And Slowly Through Your Nose

When you inhale, keep your mouth closed. Pull the air in deeply through your nose, focusing on expanding your lungs downward and pushing down on your diaphragm.

Step 3: Exhale Through Your Nose Or Mouth

Traditionally, you would exhale through your mouth, but in yoga, the way that you breathe is important. Different exhales reap different results. To slow the heartbeat and increase relaxation in a controlled way, exhale through pursed lips. To experience a nice fast release of energy, exhale in a hah sound, like a forced sigh. To improve blood flow to the brain and body, exhale through the nose with a closed mouth.[17]

Step 4: Bring Your Awareness To The Rise And Fall Of Your Hands

As you continue to breathe, pull your awareness to the rise and fall of your hands. If you notice your right hand rising, continue to pull the breath deeper into your diaphragm.

Step 5: Try To Keep A Slow Rythmic Flow Of Breath

Continue to breathe into your belly for 5-10 breaths. Maintaining a good rhythm includes either equal-length inhales and exhales or even inhales and lengthened exhales. Bring your awareness inward and take note of any sensations or shifts you feel within your body and mind.

CONSTRUCTIVE REST POSITION

There is a muscle that is often referred to as the fight-or-flight muscle because of its ability to tighten in the face of danger. It's known as the psoas muscle, and it is one of the muscles most prone to storing trauma and emotion. It is the muscle that connects the hips and lower back, with strong links to the adrenal system.[18]

The constructive rest position is a foundational somatic pose that gently allows the psoas muscle to release. It is often the base of other somatic exercises and can help restore relaxation quickly by easing the psoas muscles and taking pressure off of the heart.

Instructions

This position is one of the somatic yoga poses that you can comfortably do from bed if you'd prefer to. But finding a flat surface is ideal as it offers a better resting position for your spine.

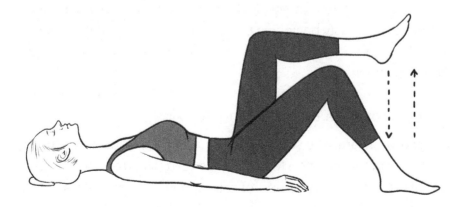

Step 1: Lie Down Flat Against The Floor

With your mat rolled out, find a comfortable resting position on your back. Make sure your spine is straight, and your head is rested in a neutral position.

Step 2: Slowly Lift The Knees And Plant Your Feet

One at a time, slowly lift each leg and plant your feet onto your mat. Your knees should be gently bent, and your feet should be hip-width apart. Keep your back relaxed without arching it or pushing it flat into the mat. Your arms should be relaxed at your sides with soft hands.

Step 3: Relax Your Body One Area At A Time

Begin to breathe deeper, using your awareness to relax your body one area at a time. You might start with your forehead, jaw, and face muscles, then slowly scan your awareness down your body until you reach your toes.

Step 4: Practice Rhythmic Breathing

As you continue to relax in this semi-supine position, bring your awareness onto your breath. Notice your natural breathing pattern before consciously beginning to deepen and lengthen it. Slow the breathing to a comfortable rhythm and use the breath to relax the body further.

Step 5: Continue Breathing And Relaxing

Keep your awareness softly on your breath and muscle softness, and relax in this position for as long as you'd like to. It can be used to release stress at the end of a long day or as a great starting position for a somatic yoga practice.

SOMATIC MEDITATION

Stress and anxiety can trigger a dissociative response where our minds disconnect from our bodies or surroundings. It can cause us to get stuck in our heads, forgetting to feel our way through trauma and emotion. Somatic meditation is a meditative practice that gently reconnects you with your body and environment. By bringing your awareness to your senses, you can tune into your body and ground yourself through intuitive movements and heightened awareness.

Instructions

Use this meditation technique to ground yourself in your daily practice or whenever you feel overwhelmed or disconnected. Start in a seated position or lie down comfortably.

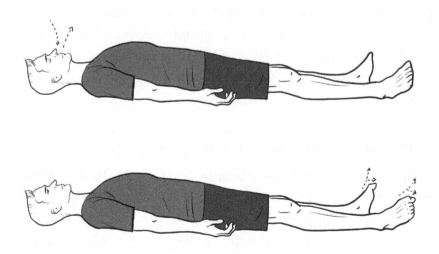

Step 1: Take A Few Deep Breaths

Begin this practice by taking a few long, slow, deep breaths down into your diaphragm. Allow the breath to center your mind into the present.

Step 2: Bring Your Awareness To Any Sensations You Feel

Gently notice where your awareness is without judgment. It may be on your thoughts, something in your environment, or a sensation in your body. As you breathe, move your awareness to any sensations you feel, even if they are uncomfortable. Just notice them without trying to change them and without lingering on them for too long.

Step 3: Keep Your Eyes Open As You Ground Into Them

Keep your eyes open as you ground your body. Use your body to shift your awareness by slowly wiggling your toes, moving your body gently, and feeling other sensations on your skin, like the wind against your face or the surface you're pressed down onto. You might choose to sway gently, stretch slowly and intentionally, or even rock back and forth in a way that feels good. Allow your eyes to fall where they want to, taking in the colors, textures, and shapes.

Step 4: As You Ground, Notice Any Shifts

With your eyes still open, continue to ground into the present moment, taking in your environment and bodily sensations. When you're ready, shift your focus back onto the sensations you felt inside your body to begin with. Notice any shifts, softening, or relief you may feel.

Step 5: Integrate With Daily Life

You can slowly shift back to your normal activities when you feel ready to. However, I will encourage you to use this practice to ground yourself during everyday tasks like eating, walking, or socializing to help you feel more present and alive in every moment.

GENTLE NECK ROLLS

The neck is a common place for stress and tension to build. It is also under a lot of strain in our modern society with the use of computers and smartphones. Neck tension can create a host of other problems, including tension headaches, brain fog, and worsened eye strain. Gentle neck rolls include variations of slow movements that stretch and relax the neck muscles.

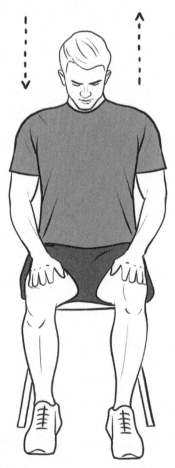

Instructions

This exercise should be done sitting up straight, starting with the neck in a neutral position. Make sure your shoulders are relaxed, and your face is forward. Keep your breath gentle, slow, and deep, inhaling through your nose and exhaling through your nose.

Step 1: Slowly Drop Your Chin To Your Chest

When you're ready, gently drop your chin to your chest, feeling the stretch at the back of your neck. Hold for 3 breaths, making sure to relax into the position.

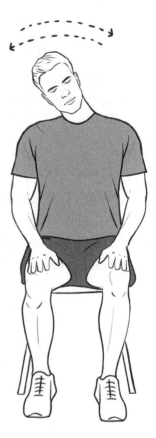

Step 2: Roll Your Neck From Side To Side

Roll your neck by keeping your chin down and slowly bringing your left ear over your left shoulder. Then, rolling back down, bring your right ear over your right shoulder. Continue rolling the neck from side to side, syncing the movement with your breath for 5-10 breaths.

Step 3: Draw A Circle In The Air With Your Nose

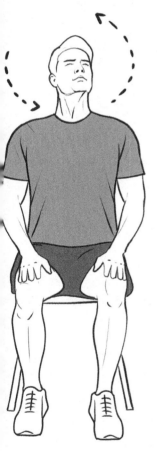

Next, progress the forward neck roll into a full neck roll by gently and slowly using your nose to draw a big circle in the air. Let your neck roll down along your chest then lift your head and look up to the sky in a full circle.

Step 4: Switch Directions And Breathe

Draw 5 circles with your nose in one direction, then switch directions and draw another 5. Make sure you are moving slowly, feeling the nice, gentle stretch as you continue to breathe and relax.

Step 5: Relax Your Neck And Slowly Lift Your Head

When you're done circling your head, rest your chin back down at your chest and completely relax there for another 3 breaths. Slowly lift your head back to a neutral position.

Step 6: Notice Any Sensations You Feel

Continue to breathe for a minute or two, taking note of any sensations you feel within your neck and head. Notice any softness, loosening, or increased bloodflow. You might feel more clear-headed or feel the need to rest for a moment.

SOMATIC YOGA NIDRA

Yoga Nidra is one of the most powerful yoga practices for a quick nervous system reset. It is a somatic meditation technique that pulls the mind and body into a blissful state of rest while awake. It is known as yogic sleep, and originates from an ancient tantric relaxation technique proven to improve wellbeing.[19] It includes body scanning, visualization, and deep inner rest.

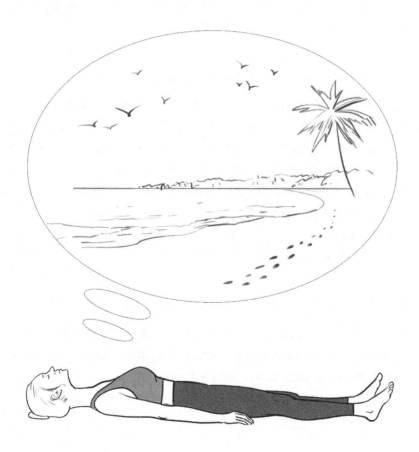

Instructions

Find a comfortable place to lie down where you won't be disturbed with arms resting next to your sides. You can lie on your mat with a blanket or do this exercise on your bed or sofa.

Step 1: Close Your Eyes And Begin With Your Tongue

You will start this exercise relaxing all the muscles in your body by pulling your awareness to each area and softening. Close your eyes and start with the muscles of your face, jaw, mouth and neck. A popular way to begin is by relaxing your tongue, then your jaw, and so on.

Step 2: Move Your Awareness Through Your Body

Breathing gently, move your awareness around your body. From your head, move down to your heart. Then, pull your awareness to the points of each arm starting with your right. Gently rest your awareness at each point for a moment. For example, rest at your shoulder, your elbow, your wrist, then each fingertip. Move it back up your arm, one point at a time, and continue down your left arm. Continue this technique down your body until you reach the tips of your toes.

Step 3: Notice Your Breath And Allow Your Body To Sink

Bring your awareness to your breath, noticing its rhythm and all the sensations included in breathing. Continue breathing deeply and slowly. Feel your body sink into the surface you're lying on with each breath. Stay present in this state of relaxation.

Step 4: Visualize A Beautiful Natural Environment

Begin to imagine yourself in a beautiful natural environment of your choosing. It could be by the ocean, in a secret garden, or next to a waterfall. Imagine all the sensations of this place, including the smells, textures, and scenery. Stay here for a moment or until you're ready to come back.

Step 5: Slowly Integrate The Experience

Start waking up from the experience, allowing the blissful state you felt in the imagined environment to stay with you. Wiggle your fingers, stretch gently, take a few deep breaths, and gently open your eyes. Keep the sensations of peace in your body to help integrate it into your reality. Practicing Yoga Nidra regularly will teach your body what peace and safety feels like.

RESTORATIVE POSES

Somatic yoga uses some of the essential practices within other yoga styles, such as yin and restorative yoga. Restorative poses are intended to open up the body, release tension, and aid in overall relaxation for the body and mind. They are simple, resting poses often accompanied by supports such as folded blankets, pillows, or yoga bolsters. Although these poses traditionally encourage full rest, allow your body to move if it will aid your relaxation.

Instructions

You can complete these poses in succession for a nice restorative somatic release of tension. Or add the poses you enjoy to your daily session as a wind-down to your practice. Use your breath to deepen poses as you relax in them for a few minutes each.

Pose 1: Supta Baddha Konasana

Also known as Reclining Bound Angle Pose, this restorative position begins on your back with feet together. Drop your knees to either side to open the hips in a butterfly position. Keep the soles of your feet together and your arms at your sides as you rest in this pose. Deepen this pose by placing a pillow underneath your knees and along the

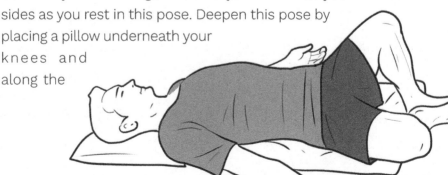

length of your spine. Then, for a somatic release of hip tension, begin to gently bounce the knees like butterfly wings.

Pose 2: Supported Child's Pose

This is a wonderfully nurturing pose that uses the body's natural comfort position. Start by kneeling on the floor with pillows or folded blankets in front of you. With a deep breath in, lift your arms up and bend forward, resting your arms and forehead on the blankets or pillows.

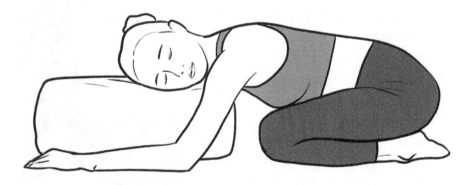

To deepen this pose, you can remove the support and rest your arms and forehead on the ground. Honor your body's needs and move it gently if you feel called to. You might roll your head from left to right for an added neck release or gently sway or rock your body.

Pose 3: Viparitha Karani

This pose releases pressure from your lower back and heart, improving circulation to the brain for a deeply calming experience. Start by lying on your back with your legs resting and extended up against a wall. Keep your arms rested at your side, allowing your body to completely surrender.

You can deepen the relaxation impact of this pose by placing a folded blanket or pillow underneath the hips to raise them slightly and underneath your head and neck. As you rest in the pose, bring your awareness to any sensations you feel. Notice any changes in your heart center, your breathing rhythm, and your state of mind. Gently release when ready. This restorative pose compliments the final exercise of this chapter greatly. Consider trying them in succession.

SIMPLE SUPINE LEG-TO-CHEST STRETCH

The lower back, hips, and hamstrings are all common places for trauma to store or tension to form. But poses don't have to involve deep stretches to be effective. One of the most effective and widely used poses to aid in relaxation, tension release, and pain management is the supine leg-to-chest stretch, also known as Apanasana.

Instructions

Find a comfortable place to lie down, preferably on a flat surface like your yoga mat on hard ground. Start in corpse pose. That is, legs down straight and your arms resting by your sides. Take a moment to deepen the breath with your eyes closed. Allow your awareness to drift around your body, taking note of any sensations or areas of interest.

Step 1: Lift One Leg At A Time And Hold

When you're ready, slowly lift the right knee towards your upper body. Interlock your hands around the knee, gently hugging it to your chest. Carefully release and repeat on the left leg.

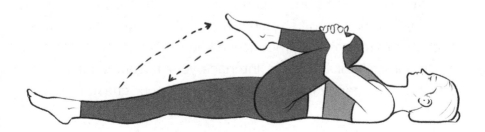

Step 2: Bring Both Legs Up And Hold

Continue this stretch by slowly lifting both knees up to the chest and gently hugging them with your arms. Hold the pose for a few deep breaths, noting the comfortable deep pressure.

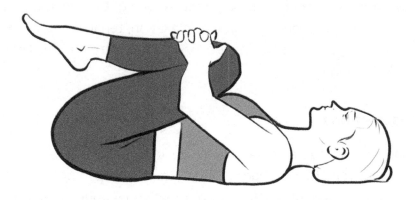

Step 3: Rock Gently From Side To Side

Still holding your knees with your arms, gently rock them from side to side, feeling the floor massage your lower back. Continue for another few breaths and release. Note any changes within your body, such as new sensations, softness, or pain levels.

Step 4: Deepen With A Hamstring Stretch

You can continue this pose if you'd like to experience a deeper hip opening and hamstring stretch. Once you're done rocking, allow both feet to rest on the ground with knees bent. Place your right ankle across your left knee. Interlace your fingers behind your left thigh and gently pull the thigh towards your chest. Feel the opening of your hips and deep stretch along your hamstring. Use the breath to soften into this position and repeat on the other leg.

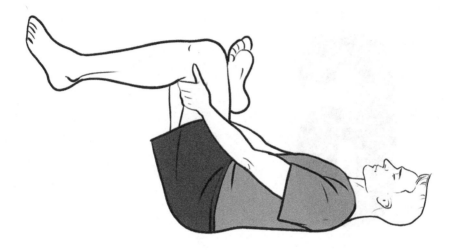

Step 5: Finish In Corpse Pose

After a couple of deep breaths, release both legs and straighten them gently along the ground. Rest your arms along your sides with palms facing up. Close your eyes and feel your body sink into the surface you're lying on. Bring your awareness to any sensations within your body. Take a couple of deep breaths while you notice any shifts, then slowly begin to move and awaken.

6

ENHANCING BODY AWARENESS AND MINDFULNESS

"How we pay attention to the present moment largely determines the character of our experience, and therefore, the quality of our lives."

— Sam Harris

BODY SCANNING

The most essential practice in somatic yoga, body scanning is a mindfulness technique that can directly improve the mind-body connection for a more regulated nervous system. By scanning the awareness through the body, this practice promotes deep relaxation, advanced present-moment awareness, and body awareness. It quickly trains your mind to understand your body and all its sensations, giving you the upper hand when shifting out of a sympathetic state. It is so essential because it forms part of many other somatic yoga exercises, deepening their impact.

Instructions

Find a comfortable place to lie down in corpse pose, with legs out straight and arms relaxed at your sides, as shown in the illustration. This is the position best used when practicing body scanning on its own, but you can incorporate a body scan into any pose or exercise for a more somatic approach.

Step 1: Begin By Centering Your Awareness

Relax your body onto the surface you are lying on, imagining it pushing up to fully support you. Take a few long, slow diaphragmatic breaths and close your eyes. When you're ready, continue to breathe deeply and center your awareness at the top of your head.

Step 2: Slowly Scan Your Awareness Through Your Body

Begin to slowly scan your awareness throughout your body, pausing along the 7 chakra points. Start at the crown of your head, then move down to the center of your head, throat, heart, solar plexus, sacrum, and the very base of your spine. Explore each area thoroughly, observing the surrounding tissue, including your arms and legs. Use the breath to deepen your awareness.

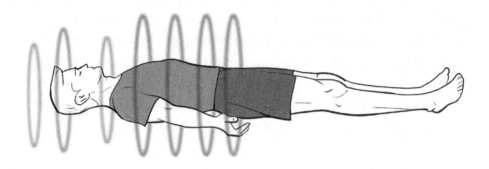

Step 3: Notice Any Sensations With Curiosity

Allow your awareness to observe any sensation you feel with a sense of curiosity. Don't try to change the sensations or avoid them. Let them be for a moment as you listen to your body's signals. They might include warmth, tingling, pressure, tension, or pain.

Step 4: Release Tension With Somatic Visualization

If there is a sensation or tension you would like to shift or release, imagine that sensation as a shape. Next, imagine a wave of cool ocean water washing over you, taking the shape with it. Imagine the shape dislodging as you consciously visualize releasing it. You can deepen the impact by consciously relaxing the areas associated with the sensation as well.

Step 5: Gently Integrate The Experience

When you're done, bring your awareness back to your breath and notice any shifts you feel. Gently integrate the experience by wiggling your toes and fingers and slowly opening your eyes.

PANDICULATION

Pandiculation is the instinctive movement pattern observed in many animals, including humans, when they wake up from a deep sleep. It includes the coordinated contraction, elongation, and release of muscles to reset the neuromuscular system for a more relaxed, tension-free body. However, in somatic yoga, we can use pandiculation to voluntarily replicate its positive effects on our neurology.

Instructions

Many movements or stretches can include pandiculation. For this exercise, I'm going to show you how you can apply the technique of pandiculation to the stretches and movements you learn. Let's use the supine leg-to-chest stretch you learned in the previous chapter as an example.

Step 1: Begin In Your Chosen Pose

Move into the pose you'd like to try pandiculation in as you normally would. For example, lying on your back, lift both knees up to your chest and hold them gently with your arms. This pose releases tension in the glutes, lower back, and parts of the psoas.

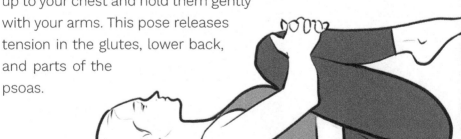

Step 2: Contract The Complimentary Muscle Systems

Next, find a way to contract the complimentary muscles of the pose you're in for about 3 breaths. For example, instead of just relaxing your knees to your chest, resist your legs against your hands. This should engage your core, hamstrings, and glutes.

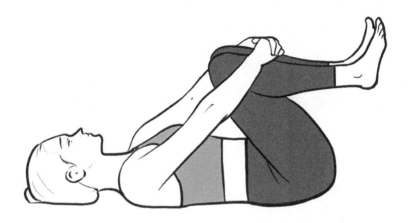

Step 3: Slowly Release The Tension And Lengthen The Muscles

Slowly release the muscles and allow them to soften into their full length. For example, allow the knees to fully relax into your chest again, feeling the hamstrings, glutes, and lower back soften.

Step 4: Notice How Pandiculation Deepens The Pose

When adding pandiculation to a pose, you should notice the pose or stretch deepen. Take note of any changes you experience. For example, after pandiculation, the supine leg-to-chest stretch should deepen, allowing your knees to soften closer to your chest.

Step 5: Take A few Deep Breaths And Repeat

Take a few deep breaths back in the normal pose and repeat. You can also alternate between a resting position before continuing with the pandiculation. For example, stretch your legs out long for a moment before lifting your knees back to your chest and repeating the pandiculation.

SENSORY AWARENESS PRACTICES

Somatic yoga relies on the 5 basic senses to ground your consciousness into the present. They include touch, sight, smell, taste, and sound. Your senses are your body's way of taking in and responding to your environment. They work closely with your nervous system to help signal important sensations to your brain. Somatic yoga often includes sensory awareness practices to help strengthen the mind-body connection and soothe the nervous system.

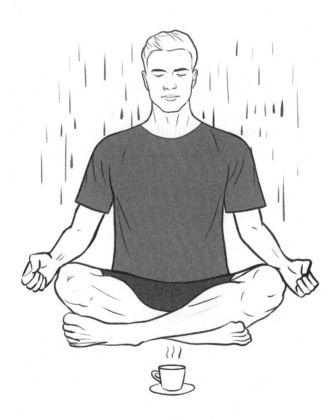

Instructions

You can incorporate these practices during and after your daily somatic practice. Use them to deepen your practice and help integrate a sense of safety and presence into daily life.

Touch Awareness

While all the senses are important, touch is one of the most impactful on your nervous system because it is the sense of your skin, which involves your entire body. The skin is the largest sensory organ. Touch awareness includes focusing on the pressure of the ground beneath you, the textures you can feel, and the temperature of the surfaces touching your body.

Sight Awareness

The eyes can take in a lot of visual details to help ground you in the present moment. In somatic yoga, sight is an important tool to help bring your nervous system out of the freeze response in particular. Rather than feeling trapped in your head, you can focus on objects, colors, and textures in your environment to pull your awareness outward.

Smell And Taste Awareness

The olfactory system of the body can trigger powerful emotional responses.[20] Trauma often stores information about smells and tastes in the brain, which is why they are a common trigger for flashbacks of traumatic events. In the same way, you can use this system to trigger states of relaxation by using smells and flavors that remind you of a safe environment. For example, you might burn a specific scented candle or essential oil during your practice to signal relaxation, such as lavender. You might choose to wear perfumes that include uplifting smells. Or, you might make a cup of relaxing tea to slowly sip on while you practice.

Sound Awareness

We've touched on the impact of vocal chord vibration on the nervous system and will cover specific exercises in Chapter 10. But you can also simply draw your awareness to sounds in your environment to help ground you into the present moment or listen to relaxing nature sounds like ocean waves, bird songs, or rain recordings, which have been proven to relax the nervous system.[21]

SOMATIC BREATH COUNTING

As you know, the breath is an integral part of somatic yoga. However, learning how to breathe deeply is not the only way to soothe the nervous system. Somatic breath counting is a mindfulness practice that uses the breath to center the mind, reduce anxiety, and improve focus.

Instructions

This exercise can be done lying down or sitting up in a meditative position. However, it can also be incorporated into almost any somatic yoga pose or during mundane activities like waiting in line at the grocery store or folding laundry.

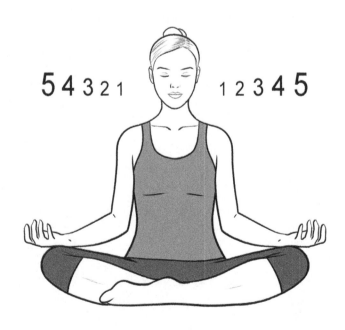

Step 1: Close Your Eyes And Focus On Your Breathing

As you get comfortable in your chosen position, close your eyes and begin to focus on your breathing without trying to change it. If you feel numb or stuck in the freeze response, keep your eyes open for this exercise, choosing something in your environment to rest your eyes on.

Step 2: Begin Counting Your Breaths

Again, without trying to change your breathing pattern, simply begin to count your breaths, counting one breath as an inhale and an exhale. There are many ways that you can count. Traditionally, you would count to 5 or 10 and repeat that sequence. However, I will encourage you to count backwards to enhance the relaxation impact of this exercise. So, count back from 5, restarting each time you reach 1.

Step 3: Maintain Your Focus

You might notice your mind begin to wander during this exercise, or you may lose track of your counting. When that happens, simply start back at 5 and continue to count down while you focus on the numbers.

Step 4: Notice Any Sensations Or Breathing Patterns

As you count, see if you can notice any natural changes in your breathing patterns or bodily sensations. You might notice your breath naturally begin to lengthen and deepen. You might notice your chest open up. Your heart rate might decrease. Or, you might notice new emotions arise. Just notice the changes for a moment.

Step 5: Repeat As Necessary

You can continue to repeat steps 2-4 for a few minutes or until you notice your anxiety and tension subside. Use this exercise whenever you feel overwhelmed, anxious, or even angry.

GROUNDING TECHNIQUES

Chronic stress is generally a result of living in a fast-paced, urban world. Our nervous systems were designed to handle major stressors out in the wild, like predators, food scarcity, and harsh weather. However, if left unmanaged, the many modern stressors we face can easily become too much. That's why regularly grounding with the earth helps to break us out of the artificial environments designed to keep us productive and remember our connection to something more.

Instructions

Grounding practices include any practice that brings your awareness to your environment. However, the most impactful grounding practices involve earthing, where your body can make contact with raw ground. Try these grounding techniques to experience earthing.

Barefoot Practice

A powerful way to earth yourself and feel grounded is to take your somatic yoga practice outdoors without shoes. Ditch the mat for this practice and allow your body to push down into the earth. Notice the sensations of your natural environment, such as the breeze, the grass, any plants nearby, or insects buzzing around. Allow your senses to immerse you in nature.

Rooting Visualization

If you can't leave your house, this technique will help you feel grounded to the earth using visualization. Simply take a moment to visualize roots growing out the bottom of your feet in any standing yoga pose. Imagine the roots reaching down into the earth and wrapping around the earth's core. You can send thoughts of love down your roots and visualize the earth responding with more love in return. This is a great practice to do at the end of your somatic yoga session to help ground you into your body. You can also practice this technique outdoors for a more profound effect.

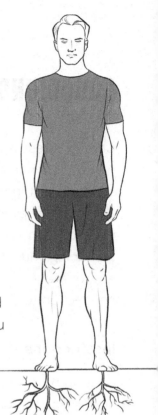

Downward Dog

Many yoga poses are great for grounding. But downward dog is one of the most effective and nourishing. To enjoy downward dog, start on the ground in a kneeling position on all fours. When you're ready, keep your hands planted firmly into the ground and allow your legs to straighten. Push into your palms, allowing your spine and hips to lift back and your head to gently relax down between your shoulders. You can see this pose in the illustration.

In downward dog, it's important to feel the points of contact you have with the ground. You can also deepen this pose by gently rocking your weight from your feet to your palms or peddling your back feet to stretch out your calves and hamstrings. Combine this with the rooting visualization for a powerful grounding somatic experience.

MINDFUL EATING PRACTICES

Eating is something we have to do every day to survive, which makes it an excellent activity for cultivating more mindfulness. It already incorporates almost all of our senses, which can be incredibly grounding. Eating is also something we do to nourish our bodies, making it a great opportunity to practice gratitude. Overall, mindful eating practices can help us find more moments of peace, joy, and well-being.

Instructions

Try these mindfulness eating practices the next time you have a meal, or try them out right now by getting a quick snack or a cup of tea. Choices with a distinct smell or flavor work very well.

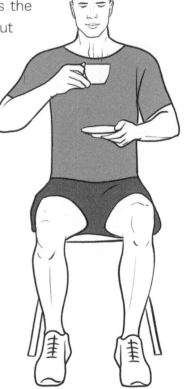

Engage Your Senses

As you prepare to eat or drink your item of choice, start to engage each of your senses. For example, if you're trying this with tea, listen to the sound that your teaspoon makes as it gently stirs against your ceramic cup. Pick the cup up and notice the warmth against your hands. Before you take a sip, bring the cup up to your nose and slowly notice any aromas. When you're ready, slowly take a sip and allow the flavors to unfold on your tongue. As you enjoy your cup of tea, take in the subtle visual aspects like the steam rising out and the design or texture of your cup. Just take it all in and allow this simple act to become a mindful sensory wonderland.

Slow Down

One of the easiest ways to practice mindfulness while eating is to slow down. Rather than sitting in front of the TV and mindlessly allowing the meal to pass, sit with the meal intentionally. Make sure that you can see your food well, focus on every bite, and fully enjoy it. Act like you're eating in slow motion to really savor the meal and practice mindfulness.

Some things you can take note of during this practice include any sensations you feel such as the texture of your food, the flavors, and other sensory input as well as the sensations of hunger and fullness you might experience. Allow yourself to experience eating as if it were the first time.

Practice Gratitude

Unfortunately, food scarcity is an issue in many parts of the world. A great way to enjoy your food more and make more mindful eating choices is to practice gratitude. You can practice gratitude in a number of ways, but simply holding a sense of giving thanks for the meal for a moment before you eat is enough. You can also set an intention for your meal to enhance the positive impact of this mindful eating practice. For example, you might set the intention, "May this meal nourish my mind, body, and spirit."

7

IMPROVING FLEXIBILITY AND MOBILITY

"Yoga must not be practiced to control the body: it is the opposite, it must bring freedom to the body, all the freedom it needs."

– Vanda Scaravelli

CAT-COW STRETCH

The cat-cow stretch is a dynamic alternation between the two yoga poses, cat and cow. It is an excellent pose for improving flexibility and mobility throughout the body as it engages almost every muscle at some point throughout the stretch. The focus on the stretch involves flexion and extension of the spine, but the somatic variation may include more spine movements.

Instructions

This is a great exercise to use when starting the dynamic portion of your somatic yoga practice. You will start on all fours and experience a great spinal warm-up. Make sure your palms are in line with your shoulders and your knees are at 90-degree angles beneath your hips.

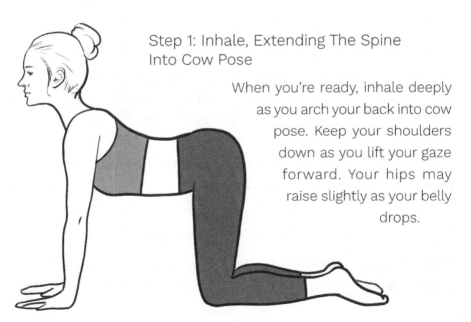

Step 1: Inhale, Extending The Spine Into Cow Pose

When you're ready, inhale deeply as you arch your back into cow pose. Keep your shoulders down as you lift your gaze forward. Your hips may raise slightly as your belly drops.

Step 2: Exhale, Flexing The Spine Into Cat Pose

Slowly exhale as you move into cat pose, gently dropping your head as you push your spine upwards and allow your pelvis to tuck in beneath you. Rest your gaze on your thighs.

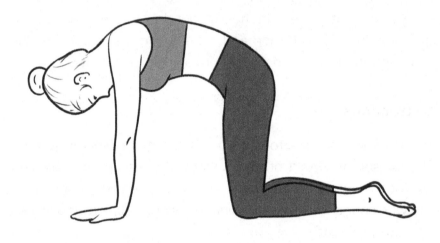

Step 3: Repeat For 3-5 Breaths, Then Hold

Continue to alternate between cat and cow, keeping your movements synced with your breath. Then, hold each pose for a few breaths. Allow your body to sink down into cow, feeling your chest open up with each breath. Then push a little deeper into cat, allowing your breath to expand your shoulder blades and your tucked pelvis to stretch your lower back.

Step 4: Begin To Move Freely Between Each Pose

Begin to sync your breath with the movements again. However, as you move between poses allow your body to shift and stretch in whichever way feels opening and releasing. You might choose to shift your weight left and right into your shoulders, gently swinging your head in the opposite direction. Or you might circle your spine as you shift between poses.

Step 5: Add A Visualization

A great visualization to try here is to imagine that you are a lion as you circle your spine between cat and cow pose. Arching your back into cow pose, you might bend your arms to drop your chest and lift your head back slightly like a lion perching on a rock. Then, as you circle your spine back into cat, you can stretch your arms down and push into your knees to deepen the pose. Notice the difference you feel in your emotions after adding the visualization.

PELVIC TILTS

Many yoga poses offer pelvic tilts for improved pelvic mobility. These poses work to release tension in the muscles that cause tightness around the pelvis. They may strengthen the pelvic muscles and help reduce pain in the lower back, hips, and hamstrings for a lasting tension release.

Instructions

Each of these poses can be included in your daily somatic yoga practice to target the pelvic region. They should all be practiced on a solid surface to reduce any strain on muscles and joints.

Pose 1: Seated Cat-Cow

The cat-cow pose offers a powerful pelvic tilt, especially when seated. Sit up straight with your legs folded and palms facing down on your knees. As you inhale, use your arms to help pull your spine gently into an arch, moving your shoulders back and lifting your gaze. Your pelvis should tilt forward, bringing your

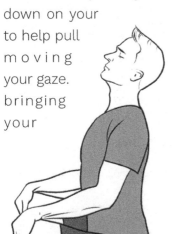

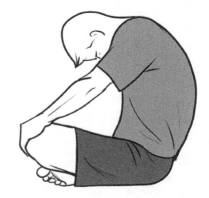

tailbone back. On the exhale, use your palms to gently extend your spine as you drop your chin to your chest and tilt your pelvis back, tucking your tailbone in. Continue to cycle between poses, keeping your breath synced.

Pose 2: Bridge Pose

Beginning on your back, bend your knees to place your feet on the mat. Rest your arms at your sides, palms pressing down gently. Slowly lift your pelvis off the ground, allowing your upper back and feet to hold your weight. This position naturally tucks your tailbone in, tilting your pelvis back. Keep your breath flowing, holding here for a moment.

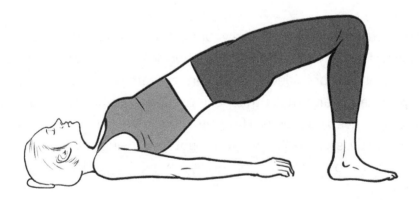

Next, slowly lower your pelvis back down and deepen with a forward pelvic tilt, arching your back slightly and bringing your tailbone back. Continue to alternate between this forward pelvic tilt, the resting position, and the pelvic lift, remembering to move slowly and intentionally.

Pose 3: Pigeon Pose

The pigeon pose is a nice challenge for a more advanced pelvic alignment. Start in downward dog, then slowly bring your left knee forward until it rests on the mat between your arms. Allow your right foot to release, resting your right knee, foot, and thigh down onto the mat.

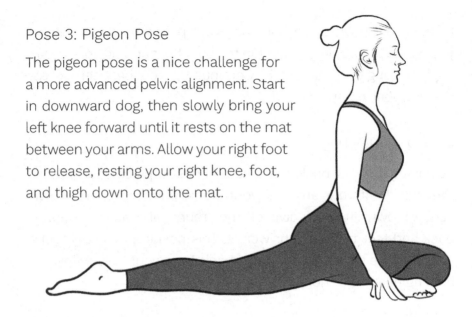

With a deep inhale, gently use your hands to lift your upper body straight, feeling your pelvis sink further down. You can use yoga blocks, pillows, or folded blankets underneath your pelvis to help lift your hands and make this pose more accessible. It is a deep stretch, so keep your breath flowing to help relax your body. When you're ready, step back onto your right foot, using your hands to push back into downward dog. Bring your left leg back and repeat on the right leg.

SPINAL TWISTS

Getting to know your spine and all the sensations along it is important for recognizing and releasing tension throughout the entire body. Spinal twists engage a wide range of muscles, improving mobility in almost every joint in the body. With each twist, you engage your shoulders, arms, head, neck, hips, and every vertebra along your spine. Spinal twists can release tension, pinched nerves, and even stimulate circulation to internal organs for improved well-being.[22]

Instructions

There are many effective positions where you can engage your body in a spinal twist. What's important is that you twist this delicate part of your body gently, using your breath and your body weight to deepen the twist rather than force. Make sure to engage your core before every twist.

Position 1: Supine Spinal Twist

Lying on your back with legs out straight and arms resting by your sides, begin to breathe deeply as you focus your awareness along the length of your spine. Inhale, lift your right knee, and place

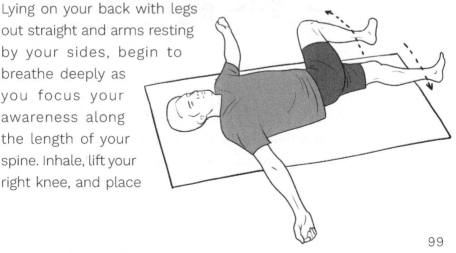

your right foot on the mat while stretching both arms up to the sky. Exhale, slowly lower your arms out to the left and right with palms facing down, as you allow your right knee to gently fall over your left leg with your head turned to the right for a full spinal twist. Hold for a few breaths, taking in the sensations along your spine, then gently release and repeat with the left leg.

Position 2: Seated Spinal Twist

In a seated position, bring your right knee up as you keep your left leg either bent or extended out straight. Hold your arms out at your sides, then gently turn your upper body, bringing your left arm over your right knee for leverage. Use your right hand on the ground behind your body and your left arm pressing against your right knee to continue the twisting motion. Gaze over your right shoulder, using your breath to slowly deepen the twist. Release gently, noticing any changes and sensations you feel along your spine, and repeat on the other side.

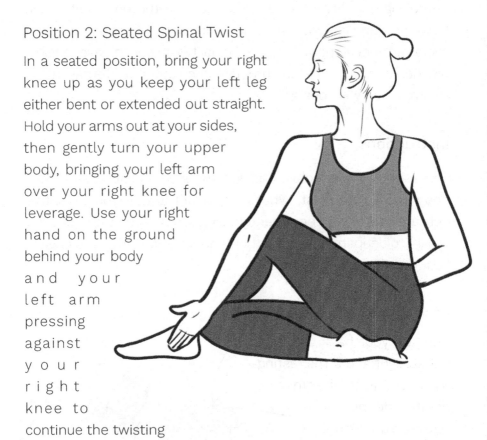

Position 3: Standing Spinal Twist

Stand up straight with your feet hip-width apart. To make this pose more challenging, you can cross your legs with a small distance between your feet. As you inhale, slowly raise your arms at either side of your body, allowing your gaze to turn and look out over your right hand. As you exhale, turn your upper body to the right, with your gaze following your right hand. Gently wrap your arms around your body and hold for 3-5 breaths.

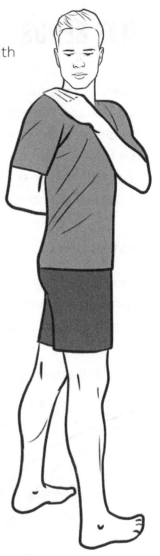

Notice any changes along your spine, such as warmth, tension, or stiffness. Use your breath to deepen the twist and release any discomfort. Carefully unwrap your arms and come back to a neutral position before repeating on the left side.

SIDE BENDS

Tension in the muscles along your torso can contribute to a host of problems, from shallow breathing to back pain. Side bends are simple bending positions that lengthen and stretch one side of the torso at a time, releasing tension throughout the entire body. They can release the intercostal muscles between your ribs, your abdominal muscles, and your hips while improving spinal mobility.

Instructions

There are many ways to execute a side bend in somatic yoga. However, the key lateral movements will remain the same for these poses as well as your somatic focus.

Pose 1: Seated Side Bend

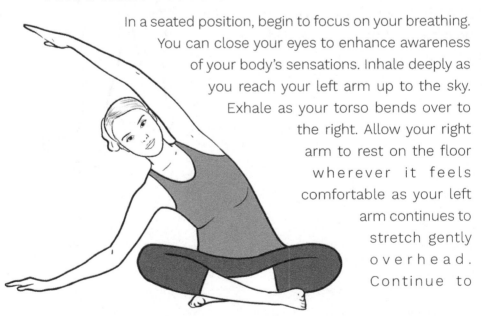

In a seated position, begin to focus on your breathing. You can close your eyes to enhance awareness of your body's sensations. Inhale deeply as you reach your left arm up to the sky. Exhale as your torso bends over to the right. Allow your right arm to rest on the floor wherever it feels comfortable as your left arm continues to stretch gently overhead. Continue to breathe deeply for a moment, feeling the muscles along your left side stretch and open. Inhale again, lifting both arms into the sky, and exhale as you switch to the other side and repeat. Continue to rest and repeat between sides in a relaxing, dynamic flow.

Pose 2: Standing Side Bend

Standing with feet hip-width apart, focus on your breathing with eyes closed to enhance awareness of the lateral movements you will be doing. Inhale deeply as you reach both arms up into the sky. As you exhale allow your right arm to slowly drop down to your right hip as you bend your torso to the right, keeping your left arm stretched overhead. Take a few breaths, noticing the sensations along your lateral body. Inhale again, stretching both arms up to the sky, and repeat on the left side as you exhale. Continue to flow between the movements, using your breath to deepen and soften the muscles along your entire torso.

Pose 3: Standing Side Bend Variation

This standing side bend variation is a little more challenging as it uses both arms to deepen the stretch and build strength in the sides of your torso. Start by standing up straight with feet hip-width apart. Inhale deeply, lifting both arms up to the sky. Clasp both hands together, keeping your arms straight over your head as you exhale and bend over to the right. Continue to breathe for a moment as you balance, hold, and feel the stretch. Inhale again, straightening your torso and lifting your clasped hands back up into the sky, keeping your arms straight throughout. Exhale again and repeat towards the other side. Notice any sensations you feel, repeating the movements in a gentle but invigorating flow.

HAMSTRING STRETCH

Many somatic yoga poses will naturally stretch out the hamstrings. However, this focused hamstring stretch allows you to rest in a pose that gently engages the hamstrings and works to release stored tension and trauma throughout the lower body. The key to successfully stretching in this pose is to relax and soften as much as possible.

Instructions

This is a seated hamstring stretch that is best practiced on a solid surface with some grip. Make sure you can take a moment to fully rest and relax without any distractions.

Step 1: Part Your Legs As Far As Comfortable

With your legs out straight, slowly part them as far as what feels comfortable, creating a wide "V" shape. Keep your toes pointing to the sky and your upper body straight.

Step 2: Focus On Your Breathing

As you feel the stretch, begin to focus on your breathing. Keep it smooth and long, deepening your relaxation. Relaxation will allow your hamstrings to fully release into this position. Close your eyes or soften your gaze, bringing your awareness to the weight of your legs on the floor.

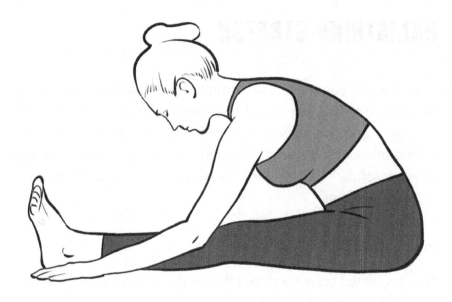

Step 3: Inhale, Folding Forward At The Hips

Allow your arms to rest gently on the floor in front of you as you inhale and bend forward. Keep your back straight and fold at the hips, feeling your hamstrings fully engage and stretch. If you can't fold down enough to rest your forearms and forehead on the floor, use pillows or folded blankets. Allow your upper body to completely relax forward.

Step 4: Breath And Relax Deeper Into The Stretch

Rest here for a moment, using your breath to deepen the stretch. As you inhale deeply, feel the expansion and stretch in your lower back. As you exhale, completely soften your entire body, allowing any tension to release. Keep relaxing, bringing your awareness to any sensations you feel while trying to keep your lower body firmly weighed down onto the floor.

Step 5: Slowly Use Your Hands To Lift Your Body

When you're ready, release from this stretch very gently. Continue to breathe as you begin pressing your hands into the ground, slowly lifting your upper body. Sit up straight, and bring your legs back to the center. You can lift your knees here, bringing your feet onto the mat and propping up your upper body with your hands behind your back. Gently drop one knee inward at a time to loosen up the inner thighs and groin area after this intensive hamstring engagement.

STANDING FORWARD BEND

Standing forward bends are incredibly beneficial for both physical and mental health. They engage the entire body, stretching the hamstrings, lower back, neck, shoulders, and arms. While releasing physical tension in the body and improving overall flexibility, standing forward bends also serve to improve confidence levels and feelings of well-being.[23]

Instructions

For this exercise, find a solid place to stand where you can fully tune into your body and relax. The somatic focus of this position includes the full backline of your body from your head to heels.

Step 1: Stand Up Straight And Breath

Stand up straight with your feet hip-width apart. Take a few deep breaths and close your eyes as you tune into your body. Bring your awareness to the backline of your body as you imagine a string pulling you from the top of your head, elongating your spine.

Step 2: Inhale, Stretch, And Fold

When you're ready to bend, inhale deeply as you stretch both arms up into the sky. Exhale, slowly bend your upper body over, folding at the hips and letting your arms reach down towards your toes.

Keep your posture good as you fold, straightening your back instead of hunching over.

Step 3: Relax Forward And Hold

Relax your upper body as much as you can, holding the pose as you breathe deeply. You can rest your hands on the ground, your shins, or you can hold your arms at the elbows for a deepened, more relaxed variation.

Step 4: Allow Movement And Focus

Begin gently swaying your upper body from left to right. Focus on how movement impacts your backline. Notice where there's tension, and use the movement with your breath to deepen and release any tension. Simply allow your body to move gently and notice the shifts.

Step 5: Gently Return To A Standing Position

When you're ready, come back to a standstill, relaxing your body down into the center again. Take another deep breath and feel the stillness in your body. Inhale, engage your core, and gently lift your upper body back up straight. You can use your hands against your thighs to help you. Inhale deeply, stretching your arms up to the sky again, elongating your entire body, and release on the exhale.

BUTTERFLY POSE

Butterfly pose, also known as Baddha Konasana, is a nourishing yoga pose for both body and mind. Serving as an excellent hip opener, stretching the inner thighs, groin, and lower back, there is a lot of tension release to experience when practicing this pose. Hip openers always include the added benefit of potentially releasing stored emotional trauma too. Allow your body and heart to open up for this pose to get the most out of it.

Instructions

This is a seated position that improves flexibility in the hips. However, if it feels a bit too challenging, you can place a pillow or folded blankets underneath the hips to soften the stretch.

Step 1: Sit Comfortably With Feet Together

In a comfortable seated position, bring the soles of your feet together in front of you. Bring your feet as close to your groin area as what feels good. It's okay if your knees are raised up here. If your knees are raised and you can't relax them comfortably, use supportive pillows or blankets.

Step 2: Hold Your Feet And Flap

Hold your feet with both hands to help steady yourself, breathing deeply to help you soften and relax. When you're ready, gently flap your knees down in a soft, bouncing motion like a butterfly flapping its wings. This should deepen the pose in a dynamic and fun way.

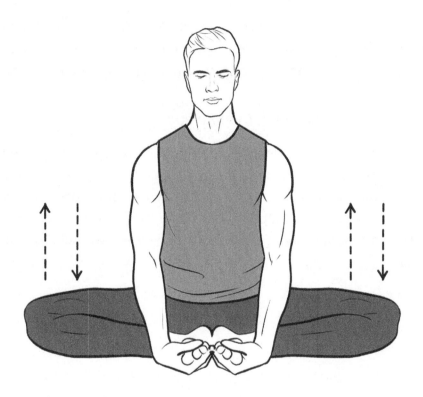

Step 3: Gently Stop Moving And Notice

Take a moment to slowly stop moving and close your eyes. Allow your awareness to float to any sensations you feel, such as tightness, warmth, tingling, emotions, or anything else. Then, try to take in the sensations of stillness that arise.

Step 4: Inhale And Fold Forward

Take a deep breath, engage your core, and as you exhale, fold your upper body forward over your feet. Use your hands holding your feet to help pull you gently into the stretch. Keep your back straight and your hips on the ground. Simply bend forward to deepen the stretch, allowing your gaze to look past your feet as if you're trying to see your reflection in a mirror on the floor.

Step 5: Relax And Hold, Then Release

Continue to take 3-5 deep breaths in this position, lengthening your spine on the inhale and leaning deeper on the exhale. Feel the stretch throughout your lower body. When you're ready, slowly engage your core to help lift your upper body back up straight. Take a moment to notice how your body feels and release the pose.

GENTLE BACKBENDS

A strong and flexible back is one of the most important assets for good mobility. Backbends are a great way to not only strengthen the muscles in your back but to release tension and blockages. Many backbends involve more advanced poses, but these 2 gentle backbends can accommodate any experience level while remaining effective.

Instructions

Make sure you have enough pillows or folded blankets to prop your weight up comfortably for pose 2. When not executed properly, backbends can put unwanted pressure on your spine, so prepare to move gently. Complete both poses on a solid, even surface.

Position 1: Cobra Flow

Begin by finding a comfortable position lying down on your stomach with legs out straight. Bring your hands underneath your shoulders and engage your core muscles. As you inhale deeply, push into your palms, lifting your shoulders gently off the ground into cobra pose, as shown in the illustration. Keep your shoulders in good posture and your gaze forward. Hold the pose for a moment as you breathe.

If lifting your upper body higher is too difficult, you can keep your body lower in baby cobra. If you'd like a challenge, lift your hips off the ground and push into the tops of your feet into upward facing dog. Feel the stretch along the muscles of your back.

When you're ready, allow your weight to rest on your forearms and palms as they face down. Press into your palms to feel your upper body expand and begin to notice the weight of your legs on the ground. Hold for 3-5 deep breaths and gently release.

Position 2: Somatic Fish Pose

Start in a seated position with legs out long and enough pillows or folded blankets to support your weight behind you. Inhale deeply, keeping your back straight. Exhale, leaning back to rest your forearms on the ground in fish pose. Close your eyes and notice the strength of your back, holding for 3 deep breaths.

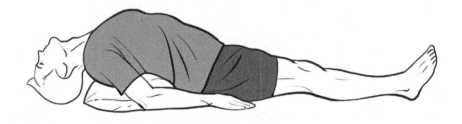

When you're ready, slowly begin to lower your weight down onto your supports. Let your upper body completely rest, allowing the supports to keep your back bent. Keep your eyes closed and feel the difference now as you relax every muscle in your body.

Notice any sensations that arise and allow your mind to rest gently on the key points of your body. With each inhale, expand your heart space, and on the exhale, allow your back to sink deeper into your supports. To finish, gently begin to wiggle your toes and fingers before opening your eyes and carefully rising out of the pose with the help of your forearms and core muscles.

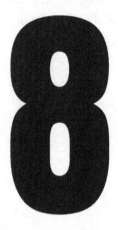

8

ENHANCING COORDINATION AND BALANCE

*"Balance is not something you find,
it's something you create."*

– Jana Kingsford

ARM CIRCLES

Mobility in the shoulders can contribute to improved blood flow in the arms and hands. It can increase your range of motion and help reduce tightness, imbalance, and pain. Arm circles are easy while offering a lot of benefits. With the somatic approach, you will also gain a new level of awareness throughout your shoulders, helping to reeducate your body to move more freely.

Instructions

This exercise can be done sitting or standing. Choose a space where you can comfortably stretch out both arms at your sides without bumping into anything. Focus on keeping your arm movements equal and balanced on both sides. Notice any imbalances in mobility and use this exercise to help even them out.

Step 1: Straighten Your Back And Raise Your Arms

Whether you are standing or sitting, make sure your back is straight and your head is in a neutral position. Bring your awareness to your shoulder sockets as you slowly raise your arms in line with your shoulders. Notice the changes in your shoulder muscles and joints as they engage.

Step 2: Begin To Circle Your Palms

Lift your palms so that your fingertips are raised to the sky, and begin to draw circles in the air with them. Keep your awareness on your shoulders and play around with the size of the circles. Expand the circles, making big, slow circles, then spiral them back into small circles. Feel the difference in your range of motion as you move.

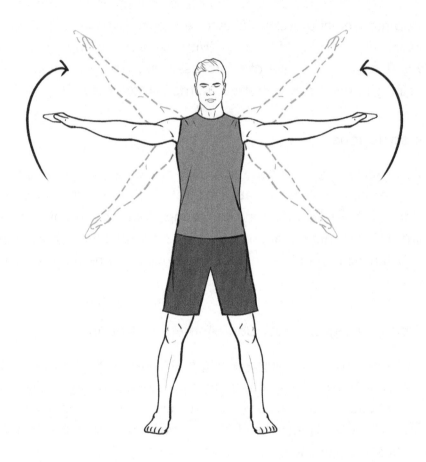

Step 3: Slow Until Still

After a few moments, begin to slow your arm circles until your arms are completely still. Take a moment to scan your shoulders and arms for any changes or sensations you can feel.

Step 4: Bend At The Elbows And Circle

Keeping your elbows in place, bring your hands to your shoulders, allowing your fingers to rest as your elbows point outwards. Focus your awareness on one shoulder at a time as you circle one elbow in a big circle. Pause, then repeat on the other shoulder. Notice the sensations, circling slowly and intentionally.

Step 5: Pause And Release

Gently slow the circling motion until your elbows are still, and unfold your arms. Allow them to soften at your sides as you pay attention to any changes and sensations you feel along the joints, muscles, and skin.

SOMATIC WALKING MEDITATION

Walking meditations are meditative walks that incorporate a deep level of mindfulness and gentle movement. They can help us feel more calm in everyday life as the practice allows us to get better at being present and relaxing even when walking around. This somatic variation combines traditional walking meditation with somatic movements to help cultivate more presence and embodiment.

Instructions

Find a quiet place where you can safely walk around, preferably outdoors. You should be able to comfortably close your eyes from time to time without bumping into anything or being in danger of falling or being hit by traffic. For added benefits, practice this meditation barefoot if the weather permits.

Step 1: Start In Standing Position With Eyes Closed

Start this exercise in a standing position and close your eyes. Begin to focus on your breathing and scan your awareness through your body. Notice any sensations you feel, slowly grounding your awareness in your body. When you reach your feet, keep your awareness here.

Step 2: Take One Step At A Time

Starting with one foot, begin to take a step forward much slower and more intentionally than you normally would. Take in all the sensations of your foot and leg as they lift. When your foot begins to touch the ground in front of you, notice every sensation from heel to toe.

Step 3: Walk Gently And Notice

Open your eyes, keeping your gaze soft, as you continue to walk gently and intentionally. Notice the sensations of your body and allow your mind to stay present. Notice what your senses pick up in your environment. Listen to the sounds, look around at the textures and colors, and see if you can smell anything.

Step 4: Add Intuitive Movements

When you're ready, begin to move more intuitively. Add arm movements, neck rolls, and anything else that feels good for your body and mind. You might start swaying gently, turn your head side to side, or gently swing your arms in an exaggerated walking posture to create soft spinal twists.

Step 5: Come To A Stand Still

After a few minutes, carefully begin to slow your movements and steps until you're standing still. Close your eyes again and focus on your breathing. Begin to scan your awareness through your body again, noticing any sensations or changes you feel. Open your eyes when you're ready.

CROSS-LATERAL MOVEMENTS

Any movements where your arms or legs simultaneously engage or cross the midline of your body are cross-lateral movements. These movements can significantly improve coordination, balance, and proprioception as they strengthen the connection between both hemispheres of the brain. They may also engage and strengthen the core muscles, which will improve balance, too.

Instructions

This exercise requires a solid floor space where your arms and hips can stay level. If the movement feels too difficult, you can use supports under your arms to raise your upper body or flip the exercise over and complete the cross-lateral movements comfortably on your back.

Step 1: Begin In Table Top Position

Start by moving down onto all fours, aligning your knees below your hips and your arms below your shoulders. Keep your back straight and balanced with your neck in a neutral position and your gaze towards the floor.

Step 2: Lift Left Arm And Right Leg

Keep your weight balanced in the center and engage your core muscles. Stretch your left arm out and forward, allowing your gaze to follow your hand. At the same time, gently lift your right leg off the ground and extend it out straight behind you. To make this pose easier, keep the knee bent.

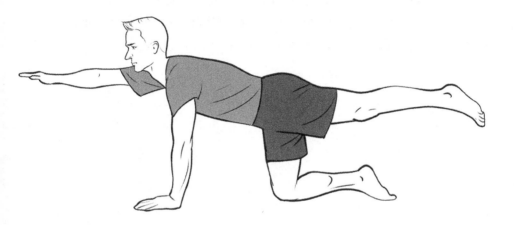

Step 3: Notice The Sensations

Take a moment to notice the sensations of keeping your balance in this position. Notice the focus it takes and which muscles are helping to keep you centered. Make sure your breath is flowing with deep diaphragmatic breaths.

Step 4: Gently Switch Arms And Legs

Slowly bring your left arm back down, pressing your palm into the mat while lowering your right knee. Allow your gaze to follow your left hand down. Gently recenter and repeat on the opposite arm and leg. You can make this pose more difficult and cross-lateral by touching your left elbow to the right knee in a cross-lateral crunch before returning to center.

Step 5: Come Back To Center

Gently return to center, pressing both palms and knees into the mat in a tabletop position. Close your eyes and take a moment to notice any sensations like warmth, stillness, or tension releasing throughout your body.

BALANCING POSES

If you've ever tried balancing with your eyes closed, you'll know how much we rely on our senses to stay upright. However, somatic balancing poses can help you balance from the core of your body through improved internal awareness and proprioception. These poses will build a sense of balance within your body, even with your eyes closed.

Instructions

Choose a solid, even surface to practice these exercises for improved balance and coordination. You can adjust the difficulty to suit your needs by using supports or adjusting the intensity.

Position 1: Tree Pose

Start in a standing position with feet together. Lengthen your back and bring your palms together at your chest. Keep your eyes open and focused on a single point in front of you as your awareness sinks into your center of gravity. Smile gently as you lift your right foot and rest it on your left leg where comfortable. You can place your foot anywhere from your left ankle to your left thigh. Allow your right knee to point to the right and hold.

If you're up for the challenge, try closing your eyes for a few seconds at a time, keeping your balance rooted. Notice the difference! After 5-10 breaths, repeat on the other leg.

Position 2: Boat Pose

Start in a seated position on the floor with the soles of your feet pressed onto the mat in front of you and your hands keeping you balanced behind you. Keeping your back straight, gently rock your torso back so your weight is pressing into your sit bones. Engage your core and focus your awareness on your center of gravity.

When you're ready, gently lift your feet off the ground. Notice the changes in your balance as your body tries not to rock back or forth. You can keep your knees bent and continue using your hands behind your back to help you balance for 3-5 breaths before resting. However, to enjoy a nice challenge, lift your arms and bring them forward in line with your legs. You can deepen this pose even further by straightening your legs with pointed toes.

Position 3: Warrior III

Start in a standing position with palms pressed together in front of your chest. Bring your awareness to your center of gravity and engage your core. When you're ready, fold at the hips, bringing your torso forward as you extend one leg back, making a T shape with your body. Keep your back straight and engaged with your gaze facing down. To increase the difficulty, reach your arms forward to extend your body more. Hold for 3 breaths, then slowly drop your leg to hinge your body up again, and repeat this on the other leg.

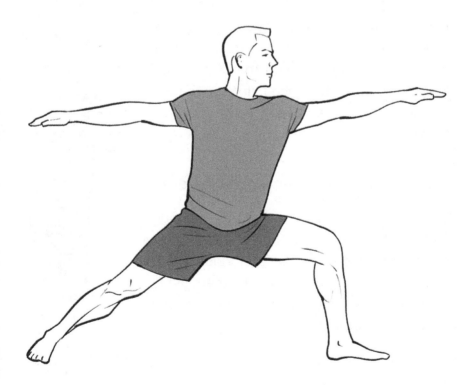

DYNAMIC STANDING POSTURES

There are many standing postures in yoga that can come together to create a nice flow of movement for a greater sense of stability and improved posture. When completed in sequence, dynamic standing postures can offer a full-body stretch or workout, improved balance, increased strength, and better mobility.

Instructions

Find a solid, even surface with enough space to extend your arms and legs out fully. Focus on moving fluidly between the poses and keeping your breath synced. If you need to balance, find a focal point in front of you to fix your gaze.

Step 1: Start In Standing Mountain Pose

Start in the standing mountain pose position with feet planted firmly into the ground at hip-width apart and arms resting at your sides. Bring your palms up to your chest, pressing them gently into each other and spreading your fingers wide for an added hand stretch.

Step 2: Stretch Up Into Upward Hands Pose

As you inhale, keep your feet firmly planted and your weight down into your legs. Keep pushing your palms together as you stretch your hands up to the sky and slightly behind you. Allow your gaze to follow the movement of your palms for a nice, controlled back bend.

Step 3: Bend Into Standing Half Moon

As you exhale, return to the center with your arms still stretched up and palms together. When you're ready, inhale and bend your torso over to the right, keeping your arms straight to deepen the side bend. Exhale and return to the center. Inhale and repeat on the other side.

Step 4: Center And Move Into Chair Pose

As you exhale and return to the center, continue to keep your arms stretched upwards. Inhale, straightening your back and lengthening your arms as you engage your core muscles. Exhale, bend your knees, and lower your hips into a seated position. Hold for a few breaths.

Step 5: Rise Up Into Upwards Hands Pose And End In Mountain

When you're ready, inhale deeply as you push your weight down into your legs and feet, rising out of chair pose and stretching up and back into upward hands pose again. As you exhale, gently return to center and lower your hands to the center of your chest. Allow your breath to flow normally again as you rest back into standing mountain. You can repeat this sequence for 3-5 rounds for a nice dynamic standing flow.

LEG LIFTS

Leg lifts help build strength and mobility in the muscles and joints of the lower body, including the hips, lower abdomen, and legs. They can also improve pelvic stability for better balance and movement efficiency.[24] A great addition to a somatic yoga practice, you can add leg lifts to your floor sessions to increase the difficulty or strength-building effects.

Instructions

Find a solid yet comfortable place to practice. You should be able to lie down on your back with your full body length extended on the ground.

Step 1: Lie Down With Legs Out Straight

Start this position in corpse pose with both legs extended out straight, allowing your body to rest completely on the floor. Allow your breath to flow deeply and slowly, focusing your awareness on your pelvic muscles and core. Engage your core as you continue.

Step 2: Lift One Leg At A Time

As you inhale deeply, slowly lift one leg off the ground, using your other leg,

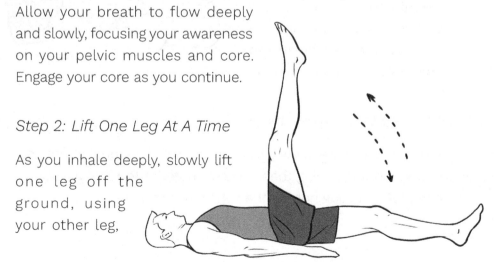

your arms, and the weight of your torso to anchor your body down. You can keep your leg slightly bent to make this pose more accessible. Exhale, gently lower your leg and repeat with the other leg. Slowly alternate lifting each leg for 5-10 rounds.

Step 3: Notice The Pelvic Sensations

As you alternate lifting your legs, keep your awareness focused on your pelvic muscles. Notice any sensations such as tightness, pain, or warmth. Notice the difficulty of the position, using your breath to help keep you steady.

Step 4: Try Double Leg Lifts

If you're up for a challenge, you can try double-leg lifts. To complete a double leg lift, press your legs and feet together and slowly lift them off the ground as you inhale deeply. Keep your body anchored down, pressing your weight into your torso, palms, and shoulders. You can hold this pose for a few breaths to challenge yourself even more.

Step 5: Slowly Lower And Rest

When you're done, slowly lower both your legs down onto the mat without dropping them. Take a moment to relax your body completely, taking note of the sensations you feel.

SQUATTING POSE

This is a position that brings us back to our body's roots, allowing us to feel balanced and grounded. Squatting the hips down into a low position may feel difficult to achieve after a lifetime of sitting in chairs, but squatting has been proven to improve health and well-being in multiple ways, including mobility and bloodflow.[25]

Instructions

If you're concerned about staying balanced or being able to squat low enough, you can use blocks or stacks of books for your hands to help you keep your upper body stable.

Step 1: Begin In Tabletop Position

Begin this position in tabletop, with knees resting in line with your hips and palms down under your shoulders. As you prepare to squat, engage your abs and start shifting your weight back.

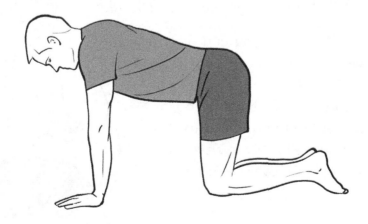

Step 2: Shift Onto Your Feet And Squat

Curl your toes under and shift your weight back until your weight is completely rested on your feet in a squatting position. Feel your hips sink down, keeping your lower back relaxed with an upright posture through your torso. Allow your knees to rest where they feel most comfortable. You can clasp your fingers together, holding your hands in front of your chest. You can also allow your hands to rest on the floor or on supports to help keep you balanced.

Step 3: Notice The Sensations In Your Lower Body

Bring your awareness to the sensations of your lower body. Notice your weight continue to sink down into your hips and onto your feet or toes. Feel the stretch along your lower back.

Step 4: Shift Your Weight From Left To Right

When you're ready, you can begin shifting your weight from the left to the right foot, feeling the gentle massage underneath your feet and through your ankles. You don't have to lift them; simply allow your weight to shift and balance over them for 3-5 breaths.

Step 5: Come Back To Center

Come back to the center, noticing how your squat has deepened since you started. Take a deep breath as you sink into the squat one last time. When you're ready, slowly drop your knees back to the mat and walk your hands forward into a tabletop position.

For an added stretch after this intensive hip opener, slowly lower your weight onto your stomach with your legs extended back. Push up onto your palms into cobra, keeping your legs flat on the ground. This should stretch the front of your hips nicely.

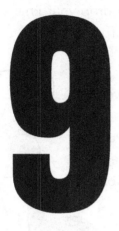

INCREASING STRENGTH AND STABILITY

"The human capacity for burden is like bamboo; far more flexible than you'd ever believe at first glance."

– Jodi Picoult

SHOULDER LIFTS AND ROLLS

All the muscles along the shoulders and shoulder blades are prone to stiffness and tension during times of stress or after trauma. We tend to hunch our shoulders or hold them in unbalanced positions, which creates imbalances in muscle strength and posture. Shoulder lifts and rolls release tension quickly and help to restore a healthy shoulder position.

Instructions

You can do this exercise sitting or standing up in a comfortable position. Just make sure you are sitting or standing on an even surface. This is a great exercise to do throughout the day when needed for a quick tension release.

Step 1: Hold Your Body With Good Posture

Stand or sit in a comfortable position, making sure that your spine is straight and your shoulders are neutral. Allow your arms to rest gently at your sides.

Step 2: Hunch Your Shoulders And Release

Begin to engage your shoulders by intentionally hunching them up towards your ears. Hold for a breath and slowly release down to a neutral position again. Emphasize the slowness of your movements for this step to give the nervous system time to release tension. Then, try to feel your shoulders elongate down without forcing them. Repeat this step 5-10 times as you breath deeply.

Step 3: Move On To Shoulder Rolls

When you're ready, move on to shoulder rolls by allowing your shoulders to rest back in a neutral position for a moment. Keep your arms relaxed at your sides, and start to roll your shoulders up, back, and down again. You can deepen the rolls by bringing them forward, then up and back, drawing full circles with your shoulders. Make sure your shoulder blades are engaged, as you imagine squeezing something between the two blades each time your shoulders roll back.

Step 4: Change Directions

After about 5-10 rolls to the back, relax your shoulders for a moment and notice any sensations you feel. When you're ready, change directions and begin to roll and circle your shoulders forward.

Step 5: Notice The Sensations

After 5-10 rolls to the front, relax your shoulders completely, feeling them soften and elongate. Bring your awareness to the sensations you feel throughout your shoulders, arms, neck, and upper back. Notice the difference in the softness and positioning of your shoulders. You might find that they are more balanced and comfortable.

HIP CIRCLES

Hip circles are a dynamic way to engage the hips for strength building and tension release. Although they may be simple, they are an excellent addition to a somatic yoga warm-up to improve blood flow, balance, and strength in the hips, side body, legs, and core. They are also a fun way to move your body, as they can feel quite silly and spark joy easily.

Instructions

This is a standing position that you can do on its own or work into many regular standing poses for added strength and stability.

*Step 1: Stand With Feet
Hip Width Apart*

Find a comfortable standing position with feet hip-width apart. You can adjust the distance between your feet to accommodate your needs or increase the difficulty. For example, standing with your feet closer together will make this exercise more challenging.

Step 2: Place Hands On Hips

Allow your hands to rest on your hips, using them to increase your awareness

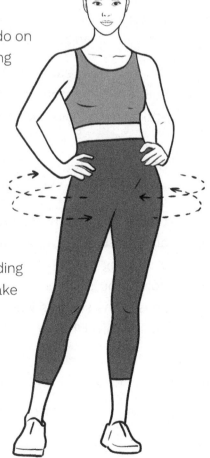

of the movements you make. Take a deep breath and continue to allow your breath to flow easily throughout this exercise.

Step 3: Begin To Circle Clockwise

Without bending your knees, draw a circle with your hips in a clockwise direction. Push them to the right, then slowly move them around to the back, then left, front, and around to the right again. Imagine you are moving a hula hoop around your torso in slow motion. You can try changing the size of your hip circles, making them bigger, smaller, or spiraling in between.

Step 4: Change Directions

When you're ready, bring your hips back to center. Notice the stillness for a moment before you continue. Begin circling in an anticlockwise direction for an equal amount of time.

Step 5: Center And Shake

After about 5-10 circles in each direction, bring your hips back to center once more. Allow your arms to rest at your sides. For an extra burst of blood flow and energy, shimmy your hips into a shaking motion for a moment. Come back to stillness and notice the suppleness of your hips, torso, and legs. Notice any sensations such as warmth, tingling, or other signs of improved energy through your lower body.

TOE AND FOOT EXERCISES

Balance starts in the toes. Your feet and toes play a major role in keeping your body upright and able to move, jump, or dance. These toe and foot yoga exercises will help improve your balance and sense of connection to the earth. They improve blood flow, flexibility, and strength in your feet, making them perfect for common toe problems and circulation issues.

Instructions

Try to complete these exercises on a solid surface, and make sure to take off your shoes and socks to connect your soles to the earth. You can use hand supports to help you stay balanced for some of these positions.

Exercise 1: Toe Squat Pose

Start in the tabletop position and tuck your toes underneath your feet. Slowly walk your hands back, pushing your hips back onto the heels of your feet. Sit up on your heels completely, feeling the stretch through your toes. You can rock your weight gently over from the left to the right foot, feeling the stretch through your toes deepen. Continue to hold and rock for 5-10 deep breaths, using the breath to help you sink your weight down into your heels, feet, and toes.

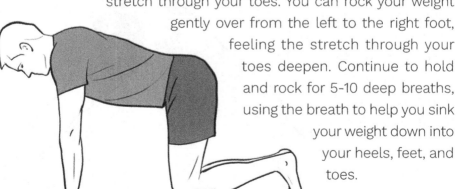

Exercise 2: Standing Toe Flexes

Stand up straight with your feet hip-width apart in standing mountain pose. Keep your body relaxed, pressing your weight down into your feet. With your feet firmly planted on the ground, try to flex your first toe on both feet as your other toes remain flat against the earth. Then, when you're ready, plant your first toe back down onto the earth and flex your other four smaller toes up to the sky. Continue to flex and rest, repeating this exercise for a few moments.

Exercise 3: Downward Dog

In tabletop position, curl your toes underneath your feet and plant your palms firmly into the ground. Straighten your legs, lifting your hips to the sky and allowing your head to drop down between your shoulders so your gaze is looking back at your feet. Keep your back straight and your feet hip-width apart or just past hip-width apart, whatever feels most comfortable. Remember to breathe deeply and slowly.

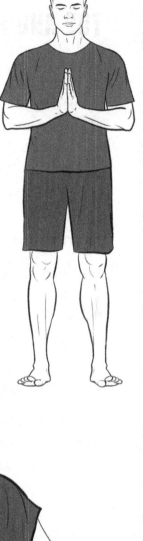

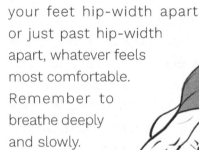

Press into your palms and the balls of your feet. Begin to bend your knees one at a time to peddle your feet against the ground. As you peddle, stretch out each foot all the way up to a pointed toe, then press the foot back down as far as what feels comfortable. This should feel like a nice strengthening massage for the feet and toes. Don't be afraid to straighten your leg and push your weight down into your heel as you peddle to make this pose more challenging.

JOINT MOBILIZATION TECHNIQUES

Every part of the body is important, from your fingers to your toes. Joint mobilization techniques aim to improve joint health and strength in a specific joint. Many of the poses you've already learned mobilize a specific joint or set of joints, such as neck rolls, hip circles, and toe squat poses. So, for these exercises, let's focus on techniques that mobilize joints otherwise neglected or difficult to reach.

Instructions

If needed, you can use supports for some of the following poses. Make sure you only deepen poses as far as you can without causing injury or putting unwanted strain on joints.

Technique 1: Finger Mobilization

This technique works to increase blood flow to the fingers for better mobility and strength. The fingers are often neglected when stretching, even though they do a lot for us. To start this stretch, sit or stand in a comfortable position and hold your hands out straight in front of you with palms facing forward. Spread your fingers as wide as they can go, as if there is a string attached to each finger, pulling it away from the palm. Slowly close your fingers into a fist and squeeze. Gently release and open the hands up again with fingers spread out. Repeat and notice the sensations.

Technique 2: Frog Pose

This technique is one of the most powerful hip-opening poses. It increases mobility in the hips by deeply improving flexibility. This is a resting pose that will open the hips more than expected, so be sure to use folded blankets or pillows underneath your hips if needed. Start in a tabletop position before bringing your feet together and widening your knees into a diamond shape.

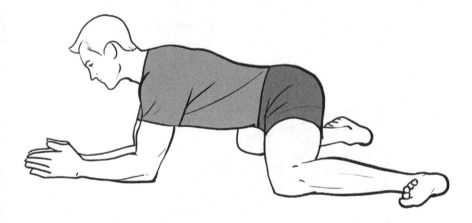

Gently stretch your arms out forward, lowering your chest towards the earth. Your weight should be pressing down into your hips as your arms help support and deepen the pose. Breathe deeply and rest into the pose for 3-5 breaths or more. When you're ready, lift your torso gently with the help of your arms and slowly move back into tabletop.

Technique 3: Plank Pose To Cobra

This flow is for improving strength and mobility in your elbows. Start in a plank position with your weight resting on your palms and toes. As you breathe, slowly lower your body down to the ground on an exhale, bending your elbows. Untuck your toes, and as you inhale, push your weight into your palms to lift your torso into cobra. Exhale, gently lowering your torso again. Tuck your toes again and inhale, pushing into your palms to lift your body back up into plank. Repeat the sequence 3-5 times, keeping your core engaged and your movements synced with your breath.

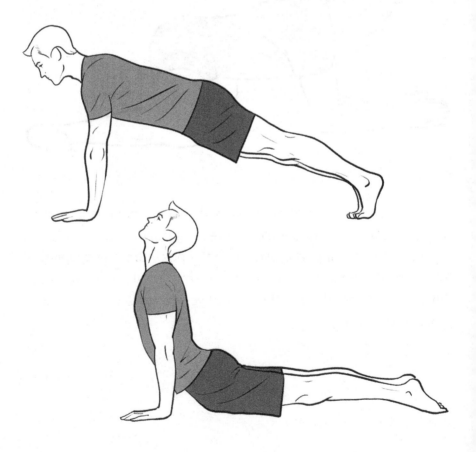

10

MIND-BODY INTEGRATION TECHNIQUES

"The partner of head is heart. Body has no opposite. In body, heart and head are one."

– Georgi Y. Johnson

BREATH AWARENESS AND MOVEMENT

Breathing patterns can influence the way we move and feel. Shallow breathing might make us feel weak or out of breath, anxious, and unwell. However, proper integration of breath with movement can help maximize your body's potential, making you feel more energized, capable, and healthy.

You've already seen breath awareness and movement in action throughout many of the other exercises and poses in the previous chapters. This exercise will help you understand how to incorporate breath awareness and movement into any pose or everyday activity. Proper breath awareness can help integrate your somatic yoga practice into life for overall improved well-being, strength, and vitality.

Instructions

Start in a standing position and prepare to experiment with various movements to practice integrating your breath with movement in the most effective way.

Step 1: Bring Your Awareness To Your Breath

In a standing position, bring your awareness to your breath. You can close your eyes and hold your left hand over your heart and your right hand over your stomach to feel the expansion of your diaphragm. Just be still here for a moment, noticing your breath and holding your awareness on the sensations.

Step 2: Use Movement To Express Your Breath

When you're ready, begin to express your breath through intuitive movement. Feel your body expand, rise, and open with every inhale. And when you exhale, feel it contract, lower, and fold. You can imagine that you are a starfish, and with every inhale, you stretch out your arms, open your chest, bend your spine gently backward, and look up toward the sky. Then, when you exhale, bend your knees and fold your arms into your chest. Hunch your shoulders in and bend your spine inwards.

Step 3: Feel The Breath Sync

Continue expanding your body with every inhale and contracting on every exhale for about 5-10 breaths. Move slowly and intentionally, breathing deeply into your diaphragm. Feel your breath sync with the movements and notice the difference in your body and mind.

Step 4: Apply This To All Movement

Begin to practice this technique with everyday movements or other somatic yoga exercises. For example, when you bend down to lift something, exhale as you bend down and inhale deeply as you lift. Use your breath as a powerful tool to keep your energy flowing and functional.

VISUALIZATION TECHNIQUES

Visualization is a powerful addition to any somatic yoga pose or practice. The mind plays a major role in the health of the body and vice versa. Combining mental exercises like visualization techniques with yoga creates a practice that can decrease tension, lower pain, and improve trauma release in a holistic and long-lasting way.

Instructions

You can incorporate these techniques into movements, complete them during your warm-up to engage your mind in the exercises or use them to wind down at the end of a session.

Technique 1: Somatic Tracking For Pain

Begin in any position that feels comfortable and start taking slow diaphragmatic breaths. Close your eyes for this exercise. When you're more comfortable, you can use them with your eyes open, too. Allow your attention to shift to any physical sensations you feel without judgment.

When you're ready, imagine any uncomfortable sensations as shapes. Use your breath to slowly dissolve the shapes as you release the sensations. You can use this whenever you'd like to deepen a pose through discomfort or help overcome a sensation in a mindful way.

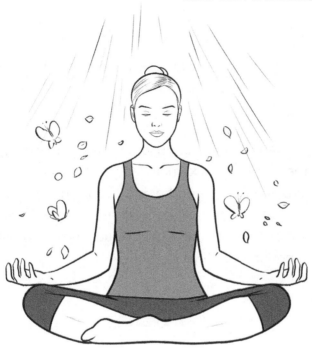

Technique 2: Breath Visualizations

In any position that feels comfortable, begin to focus on your breathing. As you inhale, visualize a white healing light entering through the top of your head, also known as your crown. Visualize this healing breath fill and move throughout your body. Allow it to pick up any stagnant energy or discomfort.

As you exhale, visualize the beautiful light exiting your nose or mouth with the energy that isn't serving you. Repeat for as many breaths as you'd like during poses, meditation, or everyday life.

Step 3: Emotion Visualization

When an uncomfortable emotion arises during your somatic yoga practice, you can use emotion visualization to address it and release it. Start by deepening your breath and bringing your awareness to the sensations of the emotion. Visualize the emotion in your body as a shape, adding details, such as texture, color, and size.

When you're ready to release it, use your breath to slowly dissolve and shift the shape. For example, as you breathe, visualize the shape getting smaller, smoother, and more beautiful. You can allow it to dissolve into sparkling dust and imagine it exiting your body through one intentional exhale. Notice the difference in your body and emotions when you're done.

SOMATIC SUN SALUTATIONS

Sun salutations are an energizing sequence of yoga poses that are traditionally done in the morning to increase blood flow and give thanks to the sun for supporting life on our planet. However, for a more gentle somatic approach, somatic sun salutations will take you through a variation of the traditional sequence in a slow and mindful way for a more peaceful practice.

Instructions

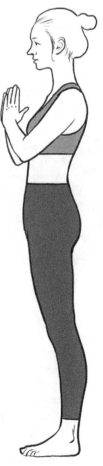

Complete this sequence on solid ground with enough grip, preferably outside or indoors, facing the direction of the sun. If completing these poses outside, make sure to soften your gaze.

Step 1: Start In Mountain Pose

Begin in a standing mountain pose with your back up straight, gaze forward, and palms pressed gently together at your chest. Spread your fingers and begin to deepen your breath. Take a moment to focus on the sensations of your body as you breathe.

Step 2: Reach Into Upwards Salute

As you inhale deeply, slowly reach up and behind your head with your palms still pressed together. Feel your chest expand, your back stretch gently, and your heart open. From this point onward, try to hold a sense of gratitude in your heart.

Step 3: Fold And Straighten Your Back

When you're ready, exhale slowly, bringing your hands back to center and folding at the hips. Allow your head to hang low, your lower back to stretch gently, and your hamstrings to engage as you balance your upper body weight down. Your arms can gently relax down to the earth, or you can hold them at the elbows for a deeper stretch. Inhale as you straighten your back into a standing half forward bend. Exhale slowly and intentionally.

Step 4: Engage Into Reverse Swan Dive

As you inhale, sweep your hands down and out at your sides like two wings as you push into your legs in a reverse swan dive. Allow your weight to anchor down as you lift your torso and continue sweeping your arms up and over your head in a controlled and intentional way. Pay attention to the opening sensation as your lungs fill with air, feeling your body come alive.

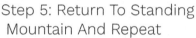

Step 5: Return To Standing Mountain And Repeat

From your reverse swan dive, bring your palms together above your head and slowly lower them back to the heart space. Steady yourself back into mountain pose and repeat the sequence 5-10 times. Remember to move slowly and intentionally, using your breath to anchor your awareness into your body. Feel your muscles engage, notice the shifts in your emotions, and be present.

SOUND AND VIBRATION

Yoga doesn't start and end with poses. Sound and vibration form an important part of a holistic somatic yoga practice that can increase the nervous system regulating impact. Whether the sound is used to engage your hearing for a more grounded mind or the vibrations are used to physically trigger the parasympathetic response, sound and vibration are useful tools at your disposal. You can use your voice or instruments to "tune" the body into a new state of being.

Instructions

I'm going to suggest a few tools you can buy or create to enjoy the benefits of sound and vibration, but your voice is all that you truly need.

Singing Bowls

These are traditionally metal or crystal bowls that you can invest in for an immersive somatic yoga experience. You can use them to open your practice, end your practice, or simply sit in meditation. A small singing bowl can be held in the palm of your hand, struck, and moved around your body to practice moving your awareness around with the sound. A DIY option includes gently tapping a spoon against a crystal wine glass filled with a bit of water or rubbing a wet finger along the top while keeping the base down flat until a sound rings out.

Mantra Chanting

Mantras such as Om have been used to raise feelings of well-being, peace, and joy since ancient times. To try the Om mantra effectively, allow your voice to deepen and repeat the word "Ohm" in a slow and lengthened way, allowing the mmmmm sound to vibrate through your throat.

There are many other mantras you can try, including English mantras, such as "I am" mantras. In these, you might simply repeat the words in a deep and melodic tone of voice, allowing them to vibrate and ring out through your throat and mouth. For example, "I am love" or "I am enough."

Humming

If you'd like to experience the nervous system balancing effects of chanting without a specific mantra, you can try simply humming different tones. Try to keep one tone for a deep exhale to feel the reverberation effectively. Deep tones are preferable for nervous system regulation.

Drumming

Slow, rhythmic drumming on a ceremonial drum can be deeply calming and even put you in a deep meditative state. If you don't have a drum, DIY options include making one out of common household items such as fabric and a container. Use a stick wrapped tightly in fabric to beat the drum for a deeper, more hearty sound.

SOMATIC DANCE MOVEMENTS

Expressing yourself through movement is a wonderful way to release tension and emotion. Somatic dance movements allow you to find flow and ease in your body by moving in ways that feel good. Of course, somatic dancing is a perfect opportunity to use music to deepen your practice. Find songs that stir your emotions in a way that encourages expression and release.

Instructions

Start in a standing position and have fun with these movements. There are no rules for somatic dancing so do what feels good. What's important is that you listen to your body.

Movement 1: Swaying With Breath

Standing with feet just past hip-width apart, begin to deepen your breath. When you're ready, soften your spine and gently begin to bend one knee at a time. Feel your body sway from left to right as you continue to breathe deeply.

You can add intuitive movements where you'd like. For example, placing your hands on your heart as you sway from side to side, closing your eyes, and lifting one foot off the ground as your weight shifts to the opposite side. Just do whatever feels good for your body or whatever movements help express your emotions.

Movement 2: Body Rolls

In a standing position with feet hip-width apart, focus your awareness on your center of gravity. As you breathe, begin to tilt your pelvis inwards and outwards gently. Allow your spine, neck, and shoulders to join into the movements, slowly rolling your spine like a wave as your pelvis tilts and rolls in and out.

You can bend your knees as needed and add other intuitive movements like wavy arm movements. This is also a great somatic dance movement to try from a seated position if you'd like to express yourself through movement while sitting. It's also a great movement to express yourself through breath, sighing, and vocalizations as your head tilts up during the body roll.

Movement 3: Improvised Dynamic Movement

Use this opportunity to fully express yourself without judgment using your entire body. Don't worry about what the movements look like. Focus only on how they feel. Allow your body to move in new ways, focusing on fluidity between movements.

Improvised dynamic movement can be fun, sensual, energizing, and freeing. Allow yourself to express your emotions through movements to fully process and release them. Add humming, chanting, or other vocalizations that naturally come up for a profound emotional release.

NADI SHODHANA

A simple yet profoundly impactful breathing technique, Nadi Shodhana, also known as alternate nostril breathing, is a great way to center the body and mind. Within a few short minutes, this technique can shift your perception to a more positive, balanced frame of mind.[26]

Instructions

Start in a comfortable seated position. This exercise can be used to begin or end your somatic yoga practice or multiple times throughout the day for an accumulative benefit.

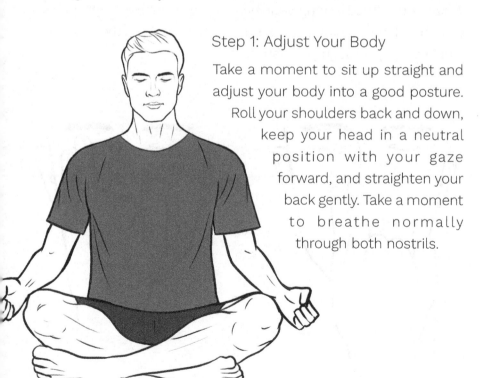

Step 1: Adjust Your Body

Take a moment to sit up straight and adjust your body into a good posture. Roll your shoulders back and down, keep your head in a neutral position with your gaze forward, and straighten your back gently. Take a moment to breathe normally through both nostrils.

Step 2: Position Your Hand Into Vishnu Mudra

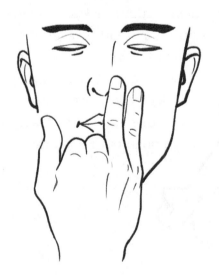

You will need to position your hand into what is known as the Vishnu Mudra, which is a hand position that will make blocking both the right and left nostrils easy. Lift your right hand so your palm is facing you. Bend your index finger and middle finger down toward the base of your thumb. Continue holding your thumb, ring finger and pinky finger out to the sides. If you find this position too difficult, you can drop your ring finger as well and use your thumb and pinky for this exercise.

Step 3: Place Thumb On Right Nostril And Inhale

When you're ready, bring your hand up to your nose and press your thumb gently down on your right nostril to block the passage. Inhale deeply through your left nostril.

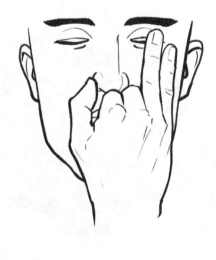

Step 4: Switch Fingers And Exhale

Pause your breath as you switch fingers. To switch, close your left nostril with your ring finger and gently lift your thumb. Exhale slowly through your right nostril.

Step 5: Inhale And Switch Fingers

Continue holding your ring finger in place, inhaling deeply through your right nostril. Then switch your fingers again, exhaling slowly through your left nostril.

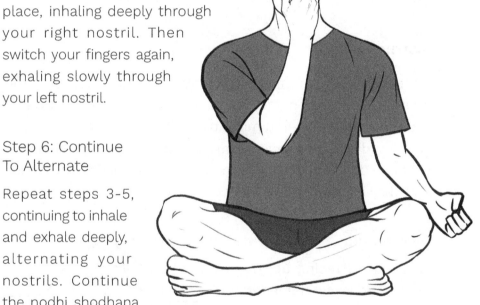

Step 6: Continue To Alternate

Repeat steps 3-5, continuing to inhale and exhale deeply, alternating your nostrils. Continue the nodhi shodhana technique for 2-5 minutes for quick and noticeable relaxing effects. This exercise may also enhance mental clarity and focus.

MUDRA PRACTICE

Mudra practice involves holding hands in various positions during meditation, everyday life, or poses to promote well-being. You've already practiced the Anjali Mudra, which involves holding hands in a prayer position, and the Vishnu Mudra during alternate nostril breathing. Allow these five additional mudras to enhance your practice.

Instructions

Deepen these mudras with somatic sensing by sensing the pressure between contact points and noticing any shifts within your body and mind. You might try adding additional pressing to your mudras or softening your mudras to gently sense the connected fingers. Try these mudras as a sequence and notice how they influence your practice.

Gyan Mudra

With palms facing up, this mudra involves touching the index finger to the thumb while keeping the other fingers extended. Hold this mudra in place for 3-5 breaths or more to aid in concentration, promote wisdom, and bring new knowledge.

Shuni Mudra

With palms facing up, this mudra involves touching the tip of the middle finger to the thumb while keeping the other fingers extended. It is practiced to promote peace, reinforce discipline, and increase focus.

Prithvi Mudra

Also known as the earth mudra, to practice prithvi mudra, hold your hand flat with palms facing up. Touch the tip of your ring finger gently to the tip of your thumb. Hold to promote increased stability, physical and emotional strength, as well as grounding.

Prana Mudra

With palms facing up, this mudra involves touching the tip of the pinky finger to the thumb while keeping the other fingers extended. Holding this mudra is said to increase vitality, energy, and life force. Try it for 3-5 breaths or more and notice any changes you feel.

Uttarabodhi Mudra

Begin this mudra with your hands in a prayer position. Press your index fingers together and your thumbs together gently. Interlace your other three fingers on both hands. Press your thumbs down, parting your palms gently. This should create a small oval of space between your thumbs and your index fingers. You can bring the mudra up above your head or rest it in your lap with index fingers pointing forward to promote self-awareness, relaxation, and spiritual growth.

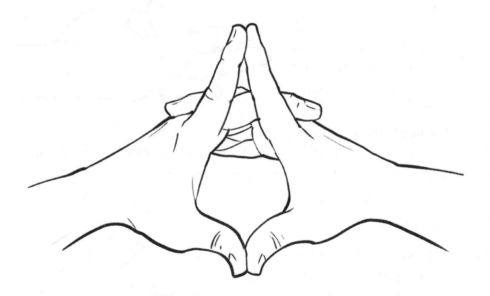

EYE MOVEMENTS

The muscles of the eyes and face are interconnected. Eye strain is a common side effect of chronic stress, tension, and overuse. Strategic eye movements can release tension built up from stress and physical exertion in the eyes, face, and scalp. You can do these eye movements as a sequence to massage and release the muscles around the head.

Instructions

Eye movements are best practiced before bed or when you can rest, as your eyes might become quite relaxed. However, you can incorporate short sequences of eye movements into somatic yoga poses or other everyday activities. Each of these exercises should be completed with good posture and your head in a neutral position, starting with your eyes gazing gently forward.

Side-To-Side Eye Movements

When you're ready, inhale as you gently and slowly move your eyes to the left as far as they can go without straining. Keep your head completely still. Hold as you exhale. Inhale again, gently and slowly moving your eyes all the way to the right without straining. Continue to move your eyes left and right, synced with your breath for 3-5 breaths. Notice where you feel the stretch.

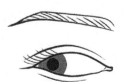
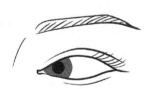

Up-And-Down Eye Movements

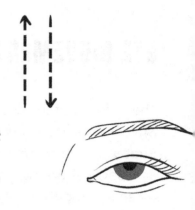

With your eyes resting forward, inhale deeply as you gently move your eyes up as far as they can go without straining. Keep your head completely still. Hold as you exhale. Inhale again, gently and slowly moving your eyes all the way down without straining or moving your head. Continue this pattern and notice the stretch for 3-5 breaths.

Diagonal Eye Movements

Imagine your up-and-down eye movements and your left-and-right movements are on an axis. With your eyes gazing up as far as they can without straining, inhale and gently roll them over about halfway to your right side. Rest them on this diagonal for an exhale. Inhale and move over to repeat on the top left diagonal. Continue this pattern to the bottom left diagonal and the bottom right diagonal, keeping the breath synced until you reach the top again.

Circular Eye Movements

When you're ready, inhale deeply as you gaze up to the sky as far as possible without straining. Exhale slowly and intentionally. As you inhale again, allow your eyes to roll in a circular motion around the entire perimeter of your gaze in a clockwise direction. Stop when you get back to the top. As you exhale, roll your eyes in the opposite direction. Repeat each time you reach the top for 3-5 breaths, remembering to move gently and slowly. Feel the stretch where it releases.

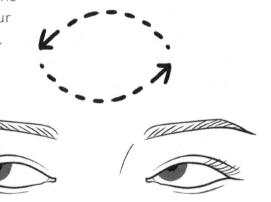

FINGER AND HAND MOVEMENTS

There are many finger and hand movements associated with yoga that can improve fine motor awareness and help your hands and fingers function more efficiently. Many yoga poses require strength and mobility in the hands, as they may end up holding a lot of weight, stretching, or assisting with balance and positioning. However, the benefits of maintaining fine motor awareness will spill off of the mat and into everyday life for years to come.

Instructions

You can complete these finger and hand exercises in a sitting or standing position. For more of a challenge, try them with your eyes closed.

Movement 1: Finger Tapping

Start by holding your left hand up with your palm facing to your right. Allow your thumb to stick out comfortably. When you're ready, take your right hand and begin to tap the fingertips of your right hand against your left thumb one by one, starting with your index finger and ending with your pinky.

You can double-tap the pinky finger and work your way back to the index finger as you repeat this pattern 3-5 times against your left hand. When you're done, switch hands and repeat against the right thumb. Take note of any changes in difficulty between sides.

Movement 2: Finger Waving

Hold both palms up in front of your
shoulders, palms facing away from you.
Start with both index fingers and work your
way out toward your pinky fingers. Bend
your index finger inward and roll it out forward,
creating an isolated wave motion with your finger.
Repeat on all four fingers, leaving your thumb flat out to the side.

Continue waving your fingers down and forward, synchronizing
your left and right hands. Repeat the pattern for about 5-10
rounds, noticing any mobility issues, stiffness, or fatigue across
your fingers.

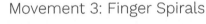

Movement 3: Finger Spirals

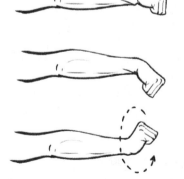

Hold both arms out straight in front
of you with palms pressed forward.
Slowly bend all your fingers in, starting
at the fingertips and rolling down into
a fist. Continue to roll, allowing your
fist to move down, bending at the
wrist. Feel the stretch throughout
your upper hand, wrist, and forearm. The
entire movement should feel like a spiral
twisting inwards.

Slowly unravel your fist and unroll your
fingers, stretching them out again. Repeat 3-5 times, focusing on
moving very slowly and intentionally. Notice any sensations such as
warmth, softness, or fatigue through your fingers, hands, and wrists.

11

INTEGRATING SOMATIC YOGA INTO YOUR LIFE

Putting The Practice To Work

"Yoga is not to be performed; it is to be lived. Yoga doesn't care about what you have been; it cares about the person you are becoming."

– Aadil Palkhivala

Somatic yoga is going to be as effective as you allow it to be. It is a powerful, ancient practice combined with one of the most impactful movement-based modern sciences for trauma release. But, much like any therapy or treatment, it won't be effective if you don't commit to it on some level. Integrating somatic yoga into your life will give it the space and time to reset your nervous system for long-term relief.

On its own, somatic yoga will create a space where you can feel safe and unwind. However, fully integrating yoga into your life could mean building a life where your nervous system always feels safe and regulated. It can make major stressors more tolerable or at least allow you to bounce back from them more effectively.

Now that you have the understanding you need let's talk about putting the practice to work. You've got the exercises at your fingertips. How do you want to bring them into your life? What will your personal somatic yoga practice look like?

Somatic yoga has enough structure to give you a powerful foundation of nervous system regulating skills without putting you in a box. It includes so much space for your unique needs. It's a practice that you can integrate into your life in a way that completely resonates with who you are. In this chapter, I'm going to recommend some lifestyle changes you can consider, somatic exercises you can use away from your mat, and some guidelines for creating your own flexible somatic yoga plan so you can get started today.

LIFESTYLE CHANGES TO SUPPORT YOUR SOMATIC PRACTICE

In our modern lives, we may become so accustomed to living in stress that we struggle to recognize the bad habits amongst the good. We might watch too much TV or choose programs that keep us on the edge of our seats. We might eat stimulating foods or drink too much coffee. We may stay up late and rob our brains of those precious hours of deep recovery sleep.

Nervous system imbalance doesn't always happen from one big stressor. It's often the little things that add up and tell our brains we aren't safe to rest.

I want you to find the peace your body is craving. It's possible to build a life that is nurturing, safe, and slow. I want you to experience that. Of course, you can't control every aspect of your life, but there is one thing you can control – your choices. You're already making choices every day that have built into the life you're currently living. Building a life that is safe for your nervous system might mean making new choices.

For a somatic practice to fully work the way you dream it will, you can't make my mistake and leave your practice at the mat. Your nervous system can't always remember peace that long. It needs reminding. That's why integrating your somatic practice into everyday life is so important. It's why embodying the beliefs and concepts of yoga can change your life for the long term.

When you create a somatically supportive lifestyle, you are constantly reminding your nervous system that it is safe. Over time, and with consistency, it can build a memory bank of safety so that eventually, even in the face of danger, it can function properly and bounce back to balance without question.

A supportive environment for your nervous system will include a holistic, integrated approach. You have to be willing to adjust your daily routine, nutrition, and mindset. The nervous system can't repair in a fast-paced, chaotic, or unhealthy environment. It needs you to commit to living your life embodying the safety it craves. You can do this by shifting:

Your Daily Routine

The nervous system needs reminders. An easy way to start shifting your lifestyle is to incorporate more moments of regulation, rest, and peace into your schedule. Two methods to continued productivity while maintaining good health and mental well-being include:

The Pomodoro Method

This is a productivity method that can help you get through the work you need to get done without burning out. You don't need to completely stop everything you're doing to factor in more rest. Sometimes, the small, frequent, bite-sized moments of rest are the most impactful.

Traditionally, the Pomodoro method would include setting a timer for 25 minutes, where you will completely focus on the task at hand, followed by a 5-minute timer for a productive break. A productive break would include getting up out of your chair to move around or stretch. It's the perfect opportunity to factor in a quick, 5-minute somatic yoga sequence or mindfulness practice.

You could also use the time to close your eyes for a quick yoga nidra power nap.

If 25 minutes to 5 minutes won't work for your schedule, you can adjust it to suit your needs. Many people apply the method to longer periods, such as 45 minutes of work followed by a 15-minute break. Just make sure you are prioritizing taking regular productive breaks rather than pushing through fatigue or stress. To try the Pomodoro method, you can set your own timer or use a Pomodoro app to help keep you on track.[27]

The Mindfulness Bell

The nervous system needs regular reminders that you are safe. Practicing mindfulness throughout the day can be an excellent way to achieve that. However, when you're caught up in your daily routine, it can be difficult to remember when to stop and ground.

A mindfulness bell can help to catch your attention and serve as a prompt to practice mindfulness. This will gently train your nervous system into a dominant parasympathetic nervous system state. It's one of the simplest ways to make calm chronic.

You can use a mindfulness bell app to set a timer for your mindfulness bell to go off. When the bell goes off, stop and take a moment to be mindful. This can include taking in your surroundings and grounding your senses, doing a quick breathing exercise, or simply checking in with your body and mind to reinforce mind-body awareness.

For a full-on approach to mindfulness, when your nervous system is feeling very dysregulated, you can set your timer to go off every 15 or 30 minutes for a couple of days to begin with. This will fast-track your mindfulness practice. However, a quick mindfulness practice every hour during your workday will make a huge difference, too.

Your Eating Habits

Your nervous system is part of your body's intricate system. Without proper nutrition, the nerves can't stay healthy or regenerate. There is no specific diet that you must follow to practice somatic yoga, but prioritizing a more nutritious diet will do wonders.

Your eating habits can also influence your nervous system state. For example, eating dinner every night in front of the TV while watching a high-energy action movie will not signal the rest-and-digest response as effectively as having a gently-lit dinner at the table with relaxing music in the background.

Food also offers many excellent opportunities to factor in mindfulness practice as it already engages all of your senses if you stay present with it. For example, when you prepare food, see it, smell it, and eat it, your senses can be fully engaged. It's something you already have to do day in and day out. Why not use it to help regulate your nervous system?

To practice mindfulness while eating, simply bring your awareness to your breathing. As you prepare your food or eat it, slow down completely and become fully present with the experience. Notice the smells, textures, colors, tastes, and sounds of the food. Simply immerse yourself in the sensory experience of eating or preparing food.

Your Sleep Hygiene

The quality of your sleep will influence every aspect of your life. It can affect your mood, energy levels, cognition, and your ability to handle stress. That's why it's often the days when we have bad sleep when we are more likely to lose our temper, become more clumsy, or feel overwhelmed.

Sleep hygiene refers to your daily habits that influence sleep, including how you spend the hours before you go to bed. Good sleep hygiene can drastically improve your sleep quality and your circadian rhythm, the internal mechanism responsible for your sleep-wake cycle. To practice good sleep hygiene, you might choose to:

- Reduce your screen time for at least an hour before bed.

- Stick to a consistent sleep schedule, going to bed and waking at the same time daily.

- Practice relaxation techniques and enjoy relaxing activities before bed.

- Keep your room cool and dark to improve comfort levels.

- Schedule your meals to avoid eating a heavy dinner just before bed.

- Limit your caffeine intake, especially in the afternoons and evenings.

- Make sure you expose your eyes to natural light first thing in the morning.

The evenings are a great time to practice somatic exercises as they may make you feel relaxed or in need of rest. However, sometimes, just one bad sleep habit is enough to create a cycle of bad sleep. So, even if you are practicing your exercises at night, consider improving your overall sleep hygiene too.

Your Activity Levels

Exercise is a great addition to any healthy daily routine. However, the type of exercise you do can impact your nervous system. If you live a high-stress lifestyle and use intense exercise to curb your stress, you may wonder why your nervous system is dysregulated even though you're exercising.

Intense exercise is not unhealthy on its own, but when you are recovering from chronic stress, it may contribute to your dysregulation by contributing to chronically high cortisol levels.[28] What your body considers intense exercise will be unique to your fitness levels. But generally, intense exercise would refer to things like high-intensity cardio or extended weight-lifting sessions.

It's up to you to gauge whether the exercise you're currently doing is contributing to your stress levels. If you think it might be, you don't have to stop completely. Perhaps just consider reducing the intensity until you're feeling more regulated.

If you're not doing any sort of exercise on a regular basis, you might want to consider adding some light, feel-good exercise into your routine. For example, you might add gentle walking, hiking, dancing, or other light forms of exercise. You might also simply include more challenging somatic yoga poses into your daily somatic yoga plan to experience a more profound endorphin release for better stress management.

SOMATIC EXERCISES BEYOND THE MAT

Along with your daily routine, there are so many powerful ways to quickly reconnect with your body. Even with a regulated nervous system, uncomfortable emotions and sensations will always find a time and a place to pop up. When they occur, it helps to have strategies in place to address them and release them without suppressing them.

Quick Somatic Exercises For Instant Stress Relief

These somatic exercises can be done anywhere and anytime to maintain and deepen the connection you're building with your body. From quick tension release to emotional processing, try them out!

Palm Press

If you work on a computer or with your hands, your shoulders might be the first place tension rises. The palm press is an easy way to release tension in the shoulder blades and upper back. To try a palm press, bring your hands together in the center of your chest in a prayer position. Inhale deeply as you press your palms together firmly. Release slowly as you exhale and relax your muscles.

You can continue to sync your press with your breath for 5-10 breaths or hold the press as your breath continues to flow for 3-5 breaths at a time.

Shoulder Shrug

A shoulder shrug is another great tension-relieving somatic exercise for shoulder pain and tightness. However, this time, the tension release is focused on your trap and neck muscles. To complete a shoulder shrug, inhale as you slowly shrug your shoulders. When you get to the top of the shrug, squeeze your shoulders toward your ears gently. Slowly release the shrug on your exhale, making sure to completely relax. Repeat for 3-5 breaths.

Box Breathing

Among the breathing exercises you've already learned, box breathing is an easy breathing pattern that can help center the mind and reduce anxiety quickly. To practice box breathing, imagine that your breathing is following a box shape with equal sides. If it helps, you can use your finger to trace the imaginary box or draw the box on a piece of paper for a more immersive experience.

To get started, inhale deeply to the count of 4. Hold your breath for the count of 4. Exhale slowly to the count of 4. Then, hold again for the count of 4. Keep repeating this pattern for a minute or two and notice any shifts in your stress levels.

Forced Yawn

Although the body is an intelligent system, it is easy to hack. In the same way that perceived stress can trigger the fight-or-flight response, the body doesn't always know what signals are authentic or not. You can follow through with forced natural processes like yawning or smiling to trick the brain into believing you are happy and relaxed.

To force a yawn, inhale deeply as you stretch your arms into the air and lengthen your back. Try to yawn when you reach the top of your inhale and exhale in a cathartic sigh as you relax your body again. Notice your body's response to a false yawn and see if you can notice any sensations similar to the real thing.

Self-Massage

Sometimes, bringing your awareness to tense areas of the body and applying some gentle self-massage techniques can make a world of difference. Self-massage allows you to offer tension relief to your muscles more readily than a once-off massage. When you feel a muscle tensing up, apply pressure with your fingers, knuckles, or the heel of your palm and experiment with different techniques to increase blood flow to the area. You can try circling motions, holding the pressure, or kneading the area.

Journaling

Emotions can run high when you're juggling the daily stressors of life. But pushing through emotions like frustration, anger, or grief without stopping to address or process them can lead to health problems down the line.[29] Journaling is an excellent somatic exercise to process uncomfortable emotions. Some journaling exercises you can try include:

- Expressive writing: The practice of writing without a filter to get your thoughts and feelings out of your body with no restrictions. You can write about something that's bothering you in a raw and unfiltered way for a quick emotional release. Give it a try in your Workbook before you continue. Choose anything that's been on your mind and let it out in the blank pages provided.

- Body scan reflection: You can use a journal to help track the sensations you feel during certain emotions to help you better identify them. Complete a quick body scan exercise while you're experiencing a strong emotion, write down the sensations, and see if you can label the emotion accurately. Writing down your reflections can help you build greater self-awareness and learn to identify your emotions before they get a chance to take over.

- Emotion expression: Express your emotions constructively through drawing, doodling, and coloring. Just like emotion visualization, you can try to express the emotion visually in your journal. Give the emotion patterns, shapes, colors, and anything else that comes through about the emotion. Expression is a powerful way to release emotional tension.

These exercises, along with many of the somatic yoga practices you've learned, are always available to help you release tension, process big emotions, or reconnect with your body during stressful times. Practicing somatic exercises during the day, even when you feel good, is the most effective way to keep your nervous system feeling safe and connected. Integrating somatic yoga into your life is the key to long-term relief.

Building A Long-Term Commitment To Your Practice

Before we move on to creating your personalized somatic yoga routine, there's one more mistake I'd like to help you avoid. We've spoken about the importance of commitment to your practice and how integrating somatic yoga into your daily life is the fastest approach to a regulated nervous system. However, with somatic exercise, it's possible to be over-committed.

The nervous system is influenced by your beliefs and thoughts. If you approach your somatic practice with a sense of urgency to feel better quickly, suddenly putting in hours of time and energy into somatic exercise and changing too much too quickly, it may backfire. That urgency to succeed might be the very thing that holds you back.

To build a long-term commitment to your practice without getting in your own way, focus on being consistent. Instead of jumping into the deep end with an intense somatic yoga workout every day, slow down and let your practice build. Set realistic goals that you can expand on, such as:

- Practice just 10 minutes of somatic yoga a day.

- Remember to be mindful throughout the day.

- Try new somatic exercises every week to find what works.

- Commit to one easy somatic exercise for quick stress relief during the day.

- Kick just one harmful lifestyle habit at a time to avoid sudden change.

Goals will help you feel motivated to actively start practicing somatic yoga so you can feel the regulation and peace that follows. To help you decide on at least one goal, complete the exercise waiting for you in your Workbook. Once you have some motivating goals in place, let's consider any obstacles that may present themselves on your yoga path.

Motivation is the biggest hurdle to climb. With the right goals, this shouldn't be an issue. However, you can add to your motivation by making sure your practice is as enjoyable as possible. If you're pressed for time or your practice space feels uninspiring, you may lose interest easily. To make your somatic yoga practice something you're itching to do at the end of a long day, I recommend:

- Choosing a practice time when you are least likely to be interrupted.

- If space is an issue, choose exercises you can do seated or from your bed.

- Try to practice outdoors to feel the freedom of unlimited space.

- Create a routine you genuinely enjoy with a good balance of exercises.

- Keep track of your progress in a journal. There is space provided in your Workbook.

- Start small so that your practice doesn't encroach on your other important tasks.

- If time is an issue, multitask by scheduling your routine during tasks that require you to wait 10 minutes or more.

For example, put your roast in the oven and set a timer, do seated exercises while you're stuck in heavy traffic if it's safe to do so, use your lunch break to practice. Start to see waiting as an opportunity to regulate yourself.

- Follow online or in-person support groups where people are passionate about the practice to help build excitement, find a sense of community, and seek guidance.

A successful somatic yoga practice doesn't require hours of commitment every week. All it takes to notice a difference is 10 minutes a day. 10 minutes is as long as it takes to microwave a meal, listen to a couple of songs, or enjoy a cup of tea.

YOUR PERSONALIZED SOMATIC PLAN – 10 MINUTES PER DAY FOR A HARMONIZED NERVOUS SYSTEM

Think of your nervous system as a balancing scale. Too much stress on one end can create dysregulation in almost any system in your body. But recovering from dysregulation isn't as simple as trying to outweigh the stress in one day of self-care.

To see a lasting difference in your nervous system's balance, you need to build up your rest-and-digest state a little bit every day. Offer your body some relief so that it knows what to expect. A consistent daily practice not only relieves tension in the moment, but it can help stop the tension from building, as you know, no matter what happens, you have the skills to cope.

Confidence in your nervous system regulating skills is enough to build a powerful resilience against stress.

Committing to just 10 minutes a day is an incredible start that will give your nervous system a great foundation to build on. It won't be long before you notice your stress levels reduce, your mood lighten, and your ability to recognize patterns of stress strengthen. A regulated nervous system won't make stress disappear, but it will make you strong enough to cope calmly.

In your Workbook, there is space to create up to 3 somatic yoga routines that you can tailor to your unique needs. You might want to create a 10-minute routine for releasing the day's stress, one for releasing long-term tension, and one for an overall nervous system reset. It's up to you what you focus on, but the formula for a well-rounded routine will be the same.

The Somatic Yoga Formula

This formula is flexible to meet your body's needs. You can adjust the timing to suit your intention. For example, you might choose to extend the amount of time you practice relaxation if your intention is to release stress, or you might choose to fill the body of your routine with resting poses rather than challenging ones. Use this as a guideline for your personalized routine.

Portion 1: Check In

Always start your routine by checking in with your body and mind. This is an important step to ensure the rest of your practice is well-suited to your needs. You can use a mindfulness exercise, a body scan, or a breathing exercise to check in.

This is also where you will choose an intention to focus on for your somatic yoga session. Your intention should match the needs you discovered during the first part of your check in. You can also choose to practice a mudra with your hands while you complete your check in for added focus. This portion of your routine should take about 1 minute and can blend into portion 2.

Portion 2: Warm Up

The next portion of your routine should involve light movements and stretches to gently engage your body. These will generally begin with your neck and upper body in a seated position. Or if you are lying down, you might choose a light hamstring stretch, lower back stretches, or arm and hand warm-ups. It should take up about 2 minutes of your routine and can be a continuation of portion one to lengthen your check-in process.

Portion 3: The Body

This portion of your routine will be heavily focused on your intention for the session. It is the body of your routine and should take up the largest portion at around 5 minutes. Depending on your intention, this portion will likely include about 3-5 somatic yoga poses. You may also choose more challenging or intensive poses that involve the whole body.

Some examples of exercises you might include here are balancing exercises, strength exercises, mobility exercises, or relaxation-focused exercises. This is a good time to practice creating a flow between your chosen poses and syncing your breath to movements.

Portion 4: Cool Down

Choose an easier exercise or two for a cool-down period of about one minute. You might choose a pose to rest into, a gentle stretch, or other relaxing exercises to bring down the intensity for a moment. Use this time to engage the body in one final movement-based exercise.

Portion 5: Integrate

It's important to end your session by integrating your experience so that you continue to feel the benefits of somatic yoga long after you roll up your mat. You might choose to integrate with another body scan, breathing exercise, or mindfulness practice. But you can also use this time to focus on your intention one last time as you practice humming, chanting, or using an instrument.

Nadi Shodhana is a great exercise to finish your practice on, or a simple Ohm mantra. You might even choose to do both! Choose an exercise that feels nourishing for both your mind and body, and gently integrate your experience before rolling up your mat and continuing with your day.

This formula is a foundation for your somatic yoga practice. It's based on a 10-minute routine, but you can adjust the timing or structure to better suit your needs. Don't let this formula limit you. Let it inspire you to build a practice that you love.

As you begin to practice, you will become more attuned to your body's needs. Keep adjusting and building your practice to work better for you as you progress. Our needs change as our bodies change. Every day is unique and brings new challenges. Use this foundation to set you up for success, and then keep going!

The nervous system doesn't bounce back from chronic stress overnight. Give your practice time to work and stay consistent. You've got all the tools you need; all that's left to do is breathe, move, and heal. Thank you for getting this far and staying committed. When you're ready, please turn the page for some final words from my heart.

CONCLUSION

Healing is a process that can feel ongoing. When you've been through a lifetime of trauma, illness, and dysregulation, being completely healed doesn't feel possible. But what does it mean to be healed?

I like to see healing as an endeavor, something to pursue as a lifelong quest. One that your spirit might continue long after it's left this body. Healing is not for broken people. It's for brave ones. It's a state that invites introspection, nurturing, and peace into your life. It's in the way that you approach your life and the things that happen while living. Healing is a way of being.

Somatic yoga contains all the power and grace of the ancient practice by which it is lovingly held. It's not intended to be separate. It's not inspired by yoga; it is yoga. Somatic elements have always been a part of yoga.

This new rendition is here to enliven what has been lost to modern yoga practice in a way that is backed by a modern, scientific understanding of our mind-body connection. Ancient practitioners already knewthese things —not in words but in wisdom. As you continue to build and deepen your practice, remember the roots of yoga and honor them.

At the heart of yoga is an ancient lineage of self-healers. Practicing somatic yoga makes you a part of that lineage.

I want to thank you for being brave enough to heal. Thank you for reaching the end of this book with the open mind it takes to recognize that everything you feel, say, think, or do is connected. I hope that what you've read has offered the next notch up in your healing journey. I hope it has stirred within you a peace that you might have forgotten or at the very least, given you the hope to continue pursuing it.

May this practice light you up as it did for me.

With love,
Rose

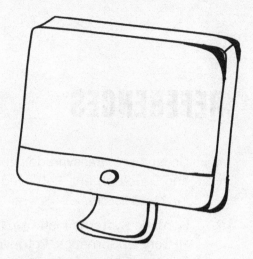

IN 90 SECONDS YOU CAN MAKE A HUGE DIFFERENCE

If you feel we've deserved it, please take a moment to leave a review on Amazon.

Your feedback means the world to us. It helps us to improve and it means better learning experiences for all our readers.

We'd be so grateful to you for your review!

Thank you!
Thank you!
Thank you!

REFERENCES

1. Dr. Ishwar V. Basavaraddi, 2015, Yoga: It's Origin, History and Development, Retrieved from https://yoga.ayush.gov.in/Yoga-History/

2. Somatic Systems Institute, 1993, A Brief Overview & History Of Somatics, Retrieved from https://somatics.org/about/introduction/overview-history

3. Andre M.M. Sousa, et al., 2018, Evolution of the Human Nervous System Function, Structure, and Development, Retrieved from https://www.ncbi.nlm.nih.gov/pmc/articles/PMC5647789/

4. Laurie Kelly McCorry, PhD, 2007, Physiology of the Autonomic Nervous System, Retrieved from https://www.ncbi.nlm.nih.gov/pmc/articles/PMC1959222/#:~:text=The%20sympathetic%20system%20controls%20%E2%80%9Cfight,%E2%80%9Crest%20and%20digest%E2%80%9D%20functions

5. Cleveland Clinic, 2022, Parasympathetic Nervous System (PSNS), Retrieved from https://my.clevelandclinic.org/health/body/23266-parasympathetic-nervous-system-psns?_gl=1*14077pe*_ga*NzAxMDc3OTIzLjE3MTI5MTY5OTQ.*_ga_HWJ092SPKP*MTcxMjkxNjk5NC4xLjAuMTcxMjkxNjk5NC4wLjAuMA

6. Callie Tayrien, RN MSN, et al., n.d., Stress Can Increase Your Risk for Heart Disease, Retrieved from https://www.urmc.rochester.edu/encyclopedia/content.aspx?ContentTypeID=1&ContentID=2171

7. Megan Riehl, PsyD, 2018, Diaphragmatic Breathing Demonstration from Michigan Medicine, Retrieved from https://www.utoledo.edu/studentaffairs/

counseling/anxietytoolbox/breathingandrelaxation.
html#:~:text=Deep%20breathing%20and%20relaxation%20
activate,oxygen%20to%20the%20thinking%20brain

8.   Alexander R. Lucas, PhD, et al., 2016, Mindfulness-Based
      Movement: A Polyvagal Perspective, Retrieved from https://
      www.ncbi.nlm.nih.gov/pmc/articles/PMC5482784/

9.   Gunjan Trivedi, et al., 2023, Humming (Simple Bhramari
      Pranayama) as a Stress Buster: A Holter Based Study to
      Analyze Heart Rate Variability (HRV) Parameters During
      Bhramari, Physical Activity, Emotional Stress, And Sleep,
      Retrieved from https://www.ncbi.nlm.nih.gov/pmc/articles/
      PMC10182780/

10.   Cleveland Clinic, 2023, Body Scan Meditation For
      Beginners: How To Make The Mind/Body Connection,
      Retrieved fromhttps://health.clevelandclinic.org/body-
      scan-meditation

11.   Ernesto Bonilla, 2008, Evidence About The Power Of
      Intention, Retrieved from https://pubmed.ncbi.nlm.nih.
      gov/19245175/

12.   Center For Clinical Interventions, n.d., Panic Information
      Sheet - 05 - Progressive Muscle Relaxation, Retrieved
      from https://www.cci.health.wa.gov.au/-/media/CCI/
      Mental-Health-Professionals/Panic/Panic---Information-
      Sheets/Panic-Information-Sheet---05---Progressive-
      Muscle-Relaxation.pdf

13.   Kayla B. Hindle, et al., 2012, Proprioceptive
      Neuromuscular Facilitation (PNF): It's Mechanisms and
      Effects on Range of Motion and Muscular Function,
      Retrieved from https://www.ncbi.nlm.nih.gov/pmc/
      articles/PMC3588663/#:~:text=Proprioceptive%20
      Neuromuscular%20Facilitation%20(PNF)%20is%20
      a%20stretching%20technique%20utilized%20to,et%20
      al.%2C%201985

14. Luiz Fernando Bertolucci, 2011, Pandiculation: Nature's Way of Maintaining the Functional Integrity of the Myofacial System?, Retrieved from https://pubmed.ncbi.nlm.nih.gov/21665102/#:~:text=Pandiculation%20is%20the%20involuntary%20stretching,rhythm%20(Walusinski%2C%20 2006)

15. Elizabeth Maria Atterbury, 2019, Exploring Therapeutic Neurogenic Tremors With Exercise As A Treatment for Selective Motor and Non-Motor Parkinson's Disease Symptoms, Retrieved from https://scholar.sun.ac.za/server/api/core/bitstreams/25662de2-756d-44ce-9ebb-e2b52792510b/content

16. Jacob Tindle, Prasanna Tadi, 2022, Neuroanatomy, Parasympathetic Nervous System, Retrieved from https://www.ncbi.nlm.nih.gov/books/NBK553141/

17. Kirsten Nunez, Cynthia Taylor Chavoustie, PMAS, PA-C, 2021, What Are The Advantages of Nose Breathing Vs. Mouth Breathing, Retrieved from https://www.healthline.com/health/nose-breathing#benefits

18. Marco A. Siccardi, et al., 2023, Anatomy, Bony Pelvis and Lower Limb: Psoas Major, Retrieved from https://www.ncbi.nlm.nih.gov/books/NBK535418/

19. Seithikurippu R. Pandi-Perumal, et al., 2022, The Origin and Clinical Relevance of Yoga Nidra, Retrieved from https://www.ncbi.nlm.nih.gov/pmc/articles/PMC9033521/

20. Elizabeth A. Krusemark, et al,, 2013, When the Sense of Smell Meets Emotion: Anxiety-State-Dependent Olfactory Processing and Neural Circuitry Adaptation, Retrieved from https://www.ncbi.nlm.nih.gov/pmc/articles/PMC3782615/

21. Hyunju Jo, et al., 2019, Physiological and Psychological Effects of Forest and Urban Sounds Using High-Resolution Sound Sources, Retrieved from https://www.ncbi.nlm.nih.gov/pmc/articles/PMC6695879/

22. Vijaya Kavuri, 2015, Irritable Bowel Syndrome: Yoga As Remedial Therapy, Retrieved from https://www.ncbi.nlm.nih.gov/pmc/articles/PMC4438173/

23. Agnieszka Golec de Zavala, 2017, Yoga Poses Increase Subjective Energy and State Self-Esteem in Comparison to 'Power Poses,' Retrieved from https://www.ncbi.nlm.nih.gov/pmc/articles/PMC5425577/

24. Lauren N. Siff, et al., 2020, The Effect of Commonly Performed Exercises on the Levator Hiatus Area and the Length and Strength of Pelvic Floor Muscles in Postpartum Women, Retrieved from https://pubmed.ncbi.nlm.nih.gov/29727372/

25. David A. Reichlen, et al., 2020, Sitting, Squating, and the Evolutionary Biology of Human Inactivity, Retrieved from https://www.ncbi.nlm.nih.gov/pmc/articles/PMC7132251/

26. Ananda Bhavanani Bhavanani, et al., 2014, Differential Effects of Uninostril and Alternate Nostril Pranayamas on Cardiovascular Parameters and Reaction Time, Retrieved from https://www.ncbi.nlm.nih.gov/pmc/articles/PMC4097918/

27. Study Lab, University of Pittsburgh, n.d., Pomodoro Technique, Retrieved from https://www.asundergrad.pitt.edu/study-lab/study-skills-tools-resources/pomodoro-technique

28. E. E. Hill, et al., 2008, Exercise and Circulating Cortisol Levels: The Intensity Threshold Effect, Retrieved from https://pubmed.ncbi.nlm.nih.gov/18787373/

29. Robert W. Levenson, 2019, Stress and Illness: A Role For Specific Emotions, Retrieved from https://pubmed.ncbi.nlm.nih.gov/31343581/#:~:text=Research%20on%20stress%20and%20disease,measured%20using%20self%2Dreport%20inventories